WINNING WITH ARTHRITIS

Harris H. McIlwain, MD
Debra Fulghum Bruce
Joel C. Silverfield, MD
Michael C. Burnette, MD

John Wiley & Sons, Inc.
New York • Chichester • Brisbane • Toronto • Singapore

Library of Congress Cataloging-in-Publication Data

Winning with arthritis / Harris H. McIlwain . . . [et al.].
    p.   cm.
    Includes bibliographical references and index.
    ISBN 0-471-52847-1
    1. Arthritis—Popular works.   I. McIlwain, Harris H.
RC933.W56   1991
616.7'2206—dc20   90-28903

Printed in the United States of America

91 92 10 9 8 7 6 5 4 3 2 1

Contributors

Frances I. Barford, L.O.T.R.

Barry C. Blass, D.P.M.

Dana S. Deboskey, Ph.D.

Ann C. Hackney, R.N., B.S.N., M.A.

Stephen F. Russell, Ph.D.

Vicki K. Winsor, R.P.T.

Acknowledgements

The authors express their deepest appreciation to these very talented individuals who helped to make this book possible:

Carol F. Bryant

Angela G. Burns

Roy E. Fulghum

Mary M. Isaac

Cordelia B. McIlwain

Linda F. McIlwain

Carole G. Reed

Pamela J. Rothman

Rick Ruge, Supervisor, Media Services, University Community Hospital, Tampa Florida

Jack R. Smith

Lori F. Steinmeyer, M.S., R.D., L.D.

Vernon L. Swenson

Kathryn H. Turner

TRADEMARKS

Advil is a trademark of Whitehall Laboratories, Inc.
AlternaGEL is a trademark of Stuart Pharmaceuticals
Alu-Cap is a trademark of 3M Riker
Alu-Tab is a trademark of 3M Riker
Amphogel is a trademark of Wyeth-Ayerst Laboratories
Anacin 3 is a trademark of Whitehall Laboratories
Anaprox is a trademark of Syntex Laboratories, Inc.
Anexsia is a trademark of Beecham Laboratories
Ansaid is a trademark of The Upjohn Company
Aristocort is a trademark of Lederk Laboratories, a division of American Cyanimid
    Company
Arthritis Strength Ascriptin is a trademark of Rorer Consumer Pharmaceuticals
Arthritis Strength Tri-Buffered Bufferin is a trademark of Bristol-Myers Products
Ascriptin is a trademark of Rorer Consumer Pharmaceuticals
Ascriptin A/D is a trademark of Rorer Consumer Pharmaceuticals
Axid is a trademark of Eli Lilly Company
Azulfidine is a trademark of Pharmacia, Inc.
Banalg is a trademark of Forest Laboratories
Bancap HC is a trademark of Forest Laboratories
Basalgel is a trademark of Wyeth-Ayerst Laboratories
Benemid is a trademark of Merck, Sharpe, & Dohme, a division of Merck & Co., Inc.
Betadine is a trademark of Purdue-Frederick Company
Capital is a trademark of Carnrick Laboratories, Inc.
Carafate is a trademark of Marion Laboratories, Inc.
Clinoril is a trademark of Merck, Sharpe, & Dohme, a division of Merck & Co., Inc.
Co-Gesic is a trademark of Central Pharmaceuticals
Cuprimine is a trademark of Merck, Sharpe, & Dohme, a division of Merck & Co., Inc.
Cytotec is a trademark of G.D. Searle & Co.
Cytoxan is a trademark of Bristol-Myers Oncology Division
Darvocet is a trademark of Eli Lilly Company
Darvon is a trademark of Eli Lilly Company
Darvon Compound is a trademark of Eli Lilly Company
Datril is a trademark of Bristol-Myers Products
Decadron is a trademark of Merck, Sharpe, & Dohme, a division of Merck & Co., Inc.
Delta Cortef is a trademark of The Upjohn Company
Deltasone is a trademark of The Upjohn Company
Depen is a trademark of Wallace Laboratories
Digel is a trademark of Schering-Plough Health Care
Disalcid is a trademark of 3M Riker
Dolobid is a trademark of Merck, Sharpe, & Dohme, a division of Merck & Co., Inc.
Duocet is a trademark of Mason Pharmaceuticals, Inc.
Easprin is a trademark of Parke-Davis
8-Hour Bayer Timed Release is a trademark of Glenbrook Laboratories
Elavil is a trademark of Merck, Sharpe, & Dohme, a division of Merck & Co., Inc.
Emperin is a trademark of Burroughs-Wellcome Company
Extra Strength Tri-Buffered Bufferin is a trademark of Bristol-Myers Products
Feldene is a trademark of Pfizer Laboratories, a division of Pfizer, Inc.
Flexeril is a trademark of Merck, Sharpe, & Dohme, a division of Merck & Co., Inc.

Gaviscon is a trademark of Marion Laboratories

Gelusil is a trademark of Parke-Davis

Hexandrol is a trademark of Organon, Inc.

Imuran is a trademark of Burroughs-Wellcome Company

Indocin is a trademark of Merck, Sharpe, & Dohme, a division of Merck & Co., Inc.

Leukeran is a trademark of Burroughs-Wellcome Company

Lorcet Plus is a trademark of VAD Laboratories

Lortab is a trademark of Russ Pharmaceuticals, Inc.

Maalox is a trademark of Rorer Consumer Pharmaceuticals

Maalox Plus is a trademark of Rorer Consumer Pharmaceuticals

Meclomen is a trademark of Parke-Davis

Medipren is a trademark of McNeil Consumer Products

Medrol is a trademark of The Upjohn Company

Metacortin is a trademark of Schering Corporation

Mortin is a trademark of The Upjohn Company

Motrin IB is a trademark of The Upjohn Company

Mylanta is a trademark of Stuart Pharmaceuticals

Mylanta II is a trademark of Stuart Pharmaceuticals

Myochrysine is a trademark of Merck, Sharpe, & Dohme, a division of Merck & Co., Inc.

Nalfon is a trademark of Dista Products Company, a division of Eli Lilly Company

Naprosyn is a trademark of Syntex Laboratories, Inc.

Nerf Ball is a trademark of Parker Brothers

Nuprin is a trademark of Bristol-Myers Products

Orasone is a trademark of Reider Rowell

Orudis is a trademark of Wyeth-Ayerst Laboratories

Panadol is a trademark of Glenbrook

Parafon Forte is a trademark of McNeil Pharmaceuticals

Pepcid is a trademark of Merck, Sharpe, & Dohme, a division of Merck & Co., Inc.

Percocet is a trademark of DuPont Pharmaceuticals

Percodan is a trademark of DuPont Pharmaceuticals

Phenaphen with Codeine is a trademark of A.H. Robbins Company, Inc.

Plaquenil is a trademark of Winthrop Pharmaceuticals

Rheumatrex is a trademark of Lederle Laboratories

Ridaura is a trademark of Smith, Kline and French

Riopan is a trademark of Whitehall Laboratories, Inc.

Riopan Plus is a trademark of Whitehall Laboratories, Inc.

Robaxin is a trademark of A.H. Robins

Roxicodone is a trademark of Roxane Laboratories, Inc.

Rufen is a trademark of Boots Pharmaceuticals, Inc.

Salflex is a trademark of Carnrick Laboratories, Inc.

Sinequan is a trademark of Roerig Division, Pfizer, Inc.

Skelaxin is a trademark of Carnrick Laboratories, Inc.

Solganal is a trademark of Schering Corporation

Soma is a trademark of Wallace Laboratories

Tagamet is a trademark of Smith Kline and Frenck Laboratories

Talacen is a trademark of Winthrop Pharmaceuticals

Talwin is a trademark of Winthrop Pharmaceuticals

Titralac is a trademark of 3M Corporation

Tofranil is a trademark of Geigy Pharmaceuticals

Tolectin is a trademark of McNeil Pharmaceuticals

Trilisate is a trademark of The Purdue Frederick Company
Tums is a trademark of Beecham Laboratories
Tylenol is a trademark of McNeil Consumer Products
Tylenol with Codeine is a trademark of McNeil Pharmaceuticals
Tylox is a trademark of McNeil Pharmaceuticals
Valium is a trademark of Roche Laboratories
Vicodin is a trademark of Knoll Pharmaceuticals
Voltaren is a trademark of Geigy Pharmaceuticals
WinGel is a trademark of Winthrop Consumer Products
Wygesic is a trademark of Wyeth-Ayerst Laboratories
Zantac is a trademark of Glaxo Pharmaceuticals
Zorprin is a trademark of Boots-Flint, Inc.
Zyclone is a trademark of DuPont Pharmaceuticals
Zyloprim is a trademark of Burroughs-Wellcome Company

Contents

CHAPTER ONE

You Can WIN!

Arthritis. It's a diagnosis over 34 million Americans heard last year. In fact, one in eight people and half of all people over the age of 65 in the United States are afflicted with arthritis. But what is this disease that causes excruciating pain and loss of the use of joints in its millions of victims? Must arthritis sufferers tolerate the constant aches that are associated with the disease? Should these people accept the immobility that accompanies their swollen, painful joints?

When Ron, age 50, came to our clinic, he told us he had been active in athletics most of his life. He played high school and college football, coached football at a large university, and was an avid golfer and tennis player. Over the last five years, he had increasing trouble playing golf and tennis because of pain in his right hip and knee. He finally stopped playing altogether.

He was examined and found to have osteoarthritis in his hip and knee. He was placed under proper medication immediately and began a specific exercise program. After two months, Ron was able to play golf and tennis without major pain. He made the decision to manage his arthritis and thereby regain his lost activities.

Nancy came to see us with symptoms very similar to Ron's. She had also been very active and enjoyed tennis and racquetball. But she had begun to develop pain and stiffness in her knees. This was followed by pain and swelling in her hands, wrists, and elbows. She developed stiffness on arising in the morning that lasted several hours and noticed fatigue after even a light workout. She also began to limit her activities gradually.

Nancy was found to have rheumatoid arthritis, and began a basic treatment program including exercises and medication. The stiffness in the morning lasted only a few minutes, and her energy returned to almost normal levels. She resumed her physical activities and began a regular swimming program.

Susan, age 32, came into our office last year, saying she was quitting her job. She reported pain and stiffness in her hands and knees, difficulty using office machines at work and even walking. After a thorough examination, Susan, too, was found to have arthritis but she chose to ignore the medications and specific exercises recommended for her condition. Today, she is unemployed and virtually disabled with constant pain in her joints.

Every day, millions of people like Ron, Nancy, and Susan are making choices regarding their arthritis. Some, like Susan, choose to accept the immobilizing pain and stiffness that arthritis brings, while others, like Ron and Nancy, choose to control these symptoms and thus live normal, active lives. This book outlines a plan for winning with arthritis, including controlling pain with special exercises, medication, and practical advice.

What Is Arthritis?

"Arthritis" means inflammation in, or around, the joints. Arthritis can attack any joint in the body: the fingers, wrists, elbows, and shoulders; hips, knees, ankles, and feet; neck, back, and other joints. The first signs of arthritis usually come on gradually but may also appear overnight. Most people feel pain or stiffness in or around one or more joints, sometimes accompanied by swelling and heat. All of these symptoms may make joints and muscles feel stiff and more difficult to use. Many people complain of feeling stiff all over on awakening. They may find that it takes time to "loosen up." Some people even lose energy and feel generally "tired all over." It may become harder to do things because of pain and stiffness in the joints. Activities that were once easy become difficult. In fact, playing golf, running, climbing stairs, walking, dressing, or even standing or writing may become gradually impossible. Arthritis related problems are among the leading causes of disability and loss of work today. 1 in every 8 of us are afflicted with some sort of arthritis!

It has been estimated that $13.1 to $17 billion in earnings are lost owing to disabling arthritis in people *under* the age of 65. People with an especially debilitating variety of arthritis, such as rheumatoid arthritis, showed earnings losses of 25 to 50 percent when compared to those with no arthritis. Some researchers found earnings losses and work disability almost as great with osteoarthritis as with rheumatoid arthritis, even though rheumatoid arthritis is usually thought to be much more severe.

There are over *100 different kinds of arthritis*. Each variety seems to behave differently and may need different treatments. The specific type of arthritis must be identified before proper treatment can be prescribed.

For example, Linda is 25 years old and had experienced six months of pain and swelling in her knees. She noticed severe stiffness in the morning on awakening, became tired easily, and had fever at night. She lost 10 pounds and began to have pain and swelling in her shoulders. Linda also started to have difficulty lifting her 2-year-old daughter. X-rays and blood tests confirmed a diagnosis of rheumatoid arthritis. Linda tried a number of medicines without improvement. She began gold injections along with exercises for the joints. After six months, her pain and swelling diminished, and she was able to perform her usual household activities including caring for her 2-year-old.

Another example was Charles, an executive, age 45, who developed severe pain and swelling in his left ankle while on a business trip so that he was unable to walk. After one week, the pain disappeared. Two months later, his right ankle and left foot became painful, swollen, and red. Even the weight of the sheets on the bed hurt his ankle and foot.

Charles was examined and a sample of fluid was removed from his ankle. This fluid was examined under a special microscope to allow a diagnosis of another type of arthritis—called gout. Treatment with a medication called allopurinol resulted in no further episodes of arthritis. A proper diagnosis allowed for specific treatment that completely controlled his pain and the disease.

Phyllis is a 50-year-old registered nurse who developed severe pain and swelling in her fingers. While she had difficulty giving patients injections and medication, no other joints were painful. Phyllis felt well except for this pain but could barely perform her duties, which required frequent use of her hands in patient care. After examination and X-rays she was found to have osteoarthritis and began regular treatments at home using a heated *paraffin bath*. She also began regular exercises to strengthen her hands and make them more limber. She was given an anti-inflammatory medication which greatly reduced the swelling and pain in her fingers. She was able to use her hands more freely and resumed her previous nursing duties.

In these examples, each person's problem required a different treatment. Linda had rheumatoid arthritis. Gold injections, which offer improvement in many patients with rheumatoid arthritis, helped her overcome her arthritis. However, gold therapy *does not work* in *all* kinds of arthritis. In gout, such as in Charles'case, allopurinol was extremely effective. Yet it would not help in rheumatoid arthritis!

Finally, Phyllis needed neither gold nor allopurinol, but used an anti-inflammatory drug with excellent results. She, therefore, was able to get effective relief without the risk of side effects from unnecessary medicines. In many cases, medication is not needed at all. These three patients are proof that you can WIN with arthritis.

Not all arthritis is the same. The idea that each type of arthritis is alike has led many people to try treatments that have no effect. The problem for someone who receives an improper diagnosis or takes ineffective medicine is that the proper treatment may be delayed at the time when it could be the most effective.

For example, Donald, at age 52, developed pain and swelling in his hands and wrists over a period of several months. He also developed pain and swelling in his ankles, knees, shoulders, and hips. He even had difficulty using his hand to open the car door, which hampered his activities as a salesman who traveled daily. He had such trouble working that he thought he might lose his job.

Then Donald heard from a friend about a clinic in another country that could cure arthritis practically overnight. Frustrated after trying several medicines, he went to the clinic where he was given unlabeled tablets. He also received injections of unknown medicines. Within a day or two, the pain disappeared in most of his joints, and he felt like a new person! He returned home but continued receiving the tablets for treatment by mail.

After a few months, Donald found his face had become swollen and round. He had gained 30 pounds but still had little joint pain. He became very ill after a minor infection and was diagnosed with diabetes mellitus requiring daily insulin injections. The tablets he had been taking for his arthritis were stopped when they were found to contain cortisone which likely allowed weight gain, infection and diabetes mellitus. After a year, he was able to stop the insulin injections. His condition was subsequently diagnosed as rheumatoid arthritis and proper treatment was given. He has now begun to lose some of the excess weight and recover from other side effects caused by the cortisone.

Sarah a 69-year-old retired teacher, was well and very active until she began to have severe pain in her right shoulder. The shoulder was so painful and stiff that she could not use her arm to comb her hair or dress in the morning. After several weeks she began to experience pain in her left shoulder as well. Sarah was seen by her physician who performed a few blood tests and diagnosed her with a type of arthritis called polymalgia rheumatica. Proper medication was administered and, within a few days, Sarah's symptoms of pain and stiffness in her shoulders disappeared.

We can conclude from these examples that there are some treatments that are very effective for certain kinds of arthritis. Some forms of arthritis can be totally controlled with certain medication, while the same medicine may have no effect on other forms of arthritis.

Take osteoarthritis, for example. The most common kind of arthritis, osteoarthritis often affects persons over 50 years old and often afflicts the knees, hips, back, and spine. These joints all contain cartilage that acts to absorb the shock of daily activities. With age, and wear and tear of daily life, the cartilage becomes

worn and does not function as well. This can result in inflammation with pain, swelling, and stiffness. With proper exercise and
treatment, persons often resume most of their lost activity.

Which is exactly what happened to Bob, a patient who is
truly winning with arthritis and controlling pain that was once
excruciating. He is a 50-year-old painter in a shipyard who began to have pain in his lower back and hips. Bob's pain became
so severe that he had difficulty standing or walking for more
than a few minutes at a time and was forced to take a leave of
absence from work. When he was examined in our clinic, he told
of his plans for early retirement due to the constant pain and
stiffness. Upon examination he was found to have typical
changes of osteoarthritis in the hips and lower (lumbar) spine.
An exercise program to strengthen his back muscles was ini-
tiated, and he adjusted his job so that he was able to avoid heavy
lifting and other excess strain on the back. After two years, Bob
continues to work full-time as a painter. The more specific the
diagnosis of arthritis, the more specific the treatment can be.
Winning with Arthritis will show you how you can help to determine which kind of arthritis you have. It is even possible for a
person to have more than one kind of arthritis. You must know
which treatments are likely to be effective and which treatments
will probably not work well. You must *avoid delay* in choosing
the correct treatment. *Winning with arthritis* and *controlling pain*
are realities if you follow the guidelines suggested in this book.
We address questions such as:

- What are important things to do in arthritis treatment?
- Does being overweight make one more likely to get
  arthritis?
- What about sports injuries? Do they increase the risk of
  arthritis in the injured joint?
- Is arthritis inherited?
- Is there a cure for arthritis or will it continue to cause pain
  your entire life?
- Can children get arthritis?
- Should a person be more active even if it hurts?
- Should one avoid any movements that actually cause pain?

When we speak of winning with arthritis, we mean managing the disease rather than "being managed" by it. There are no absolute answers to these questions. But the good news is that with an understanding of the type of arthritis, a workable program can be created including activity, rest, exercises, and medications in the proper amounts to make sure you have the maximum improvement.

If you have arthritis, then the earlier you begin treatment the better the results are likely to be. Many of the permanent changes of arthritis can be delayed or prevented if treatment is started early.

Most importantly, if you have arthritis, don't panic. Most people do not want to have arthritis and want it to go away quickly. They are very frustrated and feel they have lost control over their bodies. These are all normal feelings and need to be understood and accepted.

Attitude is one of the most important weapons to win with arthritis! And it is the one remedy that is free and has no side effects.

If arthritis is approached in an orderly way, then the confusing combination of pain, swelling, and stiffness, often with other frightening changes, can be identified. When these problems are identified and the type of arthritis is correctly diagnosed, proper treatment can begin while knowing ahead of time which treatment will have the best chances for success.

You *can* and *must* become an expert about your own type of arthritis and its treatment in order to *control pain* and *win* with the disease. You need accurate information about the cause, the available treatments, and what the future is expected to be. This book gives you this kind of information, making it possible for you to take an active part in your treatment. You can manage your arthritis in the same way you manage other areas of your life, thus allowing you to get the best possible results.

There are still no cures for most kinds of arthritis; there are no magic wands. But is very important to understand that you can learn to *control the pain* and stiffness as you manage the arthritis. With proper treatment, you can change the course of your arthritis and delay, or prevent altogether, the crippling and loss of joint use. You do not have to sit back and wait for the arthritis to take its usual course.

It is very reasonable to expect that you will eventually be able to get around and do the usual things that you would like to do in reasonable comfort. The exciting news is that *most patients can achieve this even with quite severe arthritis!* It is very unusual to see patients who cannot be helped at all, especially if the guidelines listed in this book are followed regularly.

Winning with arthritis is exactly what many people are doing. Remember, each person is different. This book cannot replace proper diagnosis and treatment for you as an individual. Talk with your physician for specific advice in your own situation.

CHAPTER TWO

The Diagnosis:
Do You Have Arthritis?

Many people wonder if they have arthritis. Most of us experience occasional aches and pains in muscles and joints. Is this arthritis and if so, which type is it? In this chapter, we discuss the symptoms and the diagnosis of arthritis.

Symptoms of arthritis include pain, swelling, or stiffness in or around the joints. There may also be warmth to the touch or redness in the skin around a joint, as well as other problems. These are signs of the inflammation that is present in arthritis.

But these symptoms are not always caused by arthritis. Soreness or pain can happen after excessive participation in yardwork, sports, or other "weekend activities." In these cases, the pain or stiffness usually goes away after a few days. The time for concern is when the pain, stiffness, swelling, or other discomfort is severe, lasts longer than a few days or returns again and again.

Arthritis Affects All Ages

Over 34 million Americans including children suffer from one or another of the 100 kinds of arthritis. The belief that arthritis is strictly an old person's disease is a myth. Arthritis is one of the most common causes of pain around the joints and muscles, and it attacks males and females of all ages.

For instance, Cathy is a 4-year-old who was seen by us recently. Her mother noticed 6 months earlier that she was irritable, especially in the mornings. When she walked in the park, she would complain that she was tired and wanted to sit down frequently. For a few months, she awakened at night with soreness in the legs that was helped by her mother's massage. Then, for a month she complained of pain in her knees and elbows. Finally, she saw her pediatrician who found no infection or other illness to explain her problems. She was found to have swelling in the knees, feet, and elbows. She began a treatment program for juvenile arthritis. Within a few months, she was almost back at her usual activity level, and participates in the same activities as her friends, including gymnastics.

In another case, Gary was a 13-year-old athlete who had been a competitive swimmer for 4 years. Over the past year, he developed pain and stiffness in his hands and feet, noticed stiffness in the morning, lost weight, and had trouble training due to fatigue. He was found to have juvenile arthritis, began a basic treatment program, and over eight to nine months experienced enough improvement in the pain, stiffness, and energy level that he returned to his previous level of competition, and continued a basic treatment program for his arthritis, including medications without any side effects.

Patients like Cathy and Gary illustrate the fact that arthritis commonly affects children as well as adults. The disease knows no barriers, attacking young and old, men and women, all races and nationalities.

Elizabeth is an 88-year-old lady who was first seen while in the hospital one week after surgery for gall bladder disease. She developed severe pain, redness, swelling, and warmth in her right first toe. She had never been bothered by arthritis before. She was unable to walk. Two days later, the same problem began in her left first toe. She was found to have arthritis caused by gout. Treatment relieved the pain and swelling in a few days, so that she was able to return to her usual activities and recover from her surgery.

John is a 72-year-old man who is a retired accountant; he is active and vigorous, playing tennis almost daily. He developed pain and stiffness in his left shoulder and was treated for bursitis. Over a few months, he began to have pain and stiffness in his hands, wrists, elbows, knees, and feet. He had swelling and warmth in the wrists and knees. He was found to have rheumatoid arthritis and began a treatment program.

Signs and Symptoms

The first signs of arthritis may develop very suddenly. Some people report that they go to bed feeling quite well and wake up with severe joint pain and swelling. More commonly, other people tell of a gradual onset of the disease, which may occur over weeks or months.

The swelling associated with arthritis may affect the joints of the hands, wrists, elbows, shoulders, hips, knees, ankles, or feet. Other joints affected may include the neck, the middle or lower back, and the jaws. Some affected persons say their pain caused them to discover joints that they never knew about!

Joan was seen by us recently because of pain in the chest. She had seen her physician and a cardiologist (heart specialist) who had found no heart disease. The pain was severe, sharp, and limited her activity. It awakened her at night. She was found to have inflammation of more than one of the small joints in the front part of the chest at the breastbone—a problem called costochondritis. She was treated and had quick improvement.

Paul is a 55-year-old man who has controlled rheumatoid arthritis. He developed hoarseness that persisted for several weeks. Because he smokes cigarettes, he was examined for throat cancer. Surprisingly, the hoarseness was found to be due to arthritis of a joint in the throat, called the *cricoaretynoid* joint.

Although we occasionally find arthritis in less common areas, certain kinds of arthritis can be expected to attack a regular pattern of joints. For example, one type of arthritis called gout has been known for more than 300 years. Usually it begins suddenly by attacking the big toe. Another type, called rheumatoid arthritis, affects many different joints in a steady, constant manner.

There continue to be questions concerning the causes of this complex disease called arthritis. For example:

- Can injuries or other illnesses cause arthritis?
- Can arthritis be inherited?
- Is there anything we can do to avoid this disease?
- Is there an immediate cure for the disease?
- What signs should alert me to begin treatment?
- Can arthritis cause death?

These are important questions. Definitive answers don't exist yet, but research is providing more and more information about the causes and treatment of many kinds of arthritis. These questions are discussed in more detail later.

Although most of us know that arthritis can cause pain and swelling in joints, there are other problems related to arthritis that are not as well-known. (See Figure 2.1.) Stiffness in the joints and muscles may be noticed upon arising in the morning. This is usually easy to feel as you notice that it takes a while to "loosen up" or "limber up." Depending on the kind of arthritis, this morning stiffness can last for hours or most of the day or it may only last a few minutes. The exact cause of the stiffness in the morning is not known. It is thought that the inactivity during sleep changes fluid in the tissues around joints to cause stiffness that gradually improves as activity increases.

This "morning stiffness" can become a potential problem for arthritis sufferers, especially for those who begin work in the morning; the stiffness may limit activity. It is common for people to adjust their entire day's schedule to accommodate this stiffness. One of our patients, an office worker, began awakening at 5 AM so that she could be more flexible and limber by 7 AM when she would leave for work. To compensate she then had to be in bed before 10 PM to get adequate sleep. Her whole lifestyle had to change to accommodate the illness.

This stiffness associated with arthritis may be quite severe or may be barely noticeable. It often worsens as the arthritis becomes more active, and usually becomes milder and lasts a shorter time as the arthritis improves with treatment.

For example, George is a 35-year-old man who works in a shipyard. He developed pain and swelling in the hands, wrists, and other joints, and found severe stiffness on awaking in the morning. The stiffness was so severe that he was able to do little work until after noon even though he began work at 7 AM. He began a treatment program for his arthritis and after 6 months he was able to "loosen up" a few minutes after a warm shower on awakening. He has continued his same job in the warehouse.

Mary is a school teacher who began to have joint stiffness and fatigue, followed within a few months by swelling and pain in the hands, wrists, shoulders, knees, and feet. The stiffness in the morning became so severe that it was difficult to bend and move around to interact as usual with her first graders. She began treatment for her rheumatoid arthritis with a regular treatment program. She improved over a few months and now is able to return to her usual level of interaction and teaching with her pupils.

Stiffness may occur at other times during the day. The troublesome feeling is almost the same as in the morning and may happen after a few minutes or longer of inactivity. This problem of stiffness during the day is sometimes referred to as "gelling." For example, sitting in one position for a period of time may make it necessary to loosen up again. This may happen after sitting in church for an hour, sitting in a classroom, or sitting at a typewriter or word processor at work. This problem of stiffness can happen anytime there is inactivity. Many people with arthritis, therefore, do best if they keep some level of activity throughout the day. In other words, it is common for arthritis patients to feel worse with too much rest as well as with too much activity!

John is a 68-year-old man who over a few weeks began to have severe pain and stiffness in his shoulders, arms, thighs, and hips. He had severe stiffness in the morning on arising and had difficulty sleeping at night due to pain. He found he needed the help of his wife to turn over in bed. He had no joint swelling. He was found to have inflammatory arthritis and improved after a few days of treatment.

Although these examples are problems caused by arthritis, the treatment and subsequent improvement follow entirely different paths.

Some Common Joint Problems in Arthritis

Joint Pain   Joint Warmth
Joint Swelling   Joint Redness
Joint Stiffness

Some Problems Other Than Joint Pain in Arthritis

Stiffness in the morning on arising   Lung disease
Fatigue   Kidney disease
Weight Loss   Shortness of breath
Fever   Difficulty swallowing
Rash   Headache
Discoloration of the fingers on cold   Hypertension
  exposure   Seizures
Sensitivity to the sun   Genital ulcers
Loss of hair   Painful urination
Mouth ulcers   Diarrhea
Back pain   Vision changes
Neck pain   Eye inflammation
Eye dryness and loss of vision   Sinusitis
Chest pain   Liver disease
Heart disease   Abdominal pain

Figure 2.1.   Common problems.

Fatigue—A Common Problem

Fatigue is a common problem many persons experience with arthritis. This fatigue may be dominant and overwhelming, and it actually may be more limiting than the joint pain and swelling in arthritis. Many people claim that if only their fatigue and lack of energy could be improved, then they could live with their joint pain and swelling.

Susan is 36 and was seen recently with joint pain, stiffness and swelling. She was found to have rheumatoid arthritis. She was bothered most by severe fatigue that limited her work in sales, which required traveling.

She considered changing jobs because of the fatigue but after her arthritis responded to treatment, her fatigue improved as well as her joint pain and swelling. She has resumed her usual level of traveling without limitation.

There are many other causes of fatigue. It is important to be sure that problems other than arthritis are found and corrected. If no other problems are present, fatigue can often be explained as part of the arthritis just as the more obvious swelling in joints.

Fatigue may make a person appear to be lazy or poorly motivated. Family, friends, or employers may feel the person doesn't care or isn't trying as hard as before. If this symptom is not identified and treated, then problems with family and work relations may cause severe misunderstanding and stress.

Fatigue is probably the most difficult symptom to understand for those who don't have arthritis. It may be especially hard on family members who see their relative become less active and require more rest. When this happens with a mother or father, it can be devastating to a family. One way of understanding what the fatigue of arthritis is like may be to remember the last time you suffered with the "flu" or similar illness. The feeling of extreme fatigue and lack of energy probably lasted a few days. Try to imagine this feeling being present *all of the time.* This is somewhat like the feeling many arthritis patients have each day.

The good news is that the fatigue usually improves as the arthritis gets better with treatment, although it may be slower to respond than the joint pain or swelling.

Not all kinds of arthritis bring severe fatigue, just as not all kinds of arthritis have stiffness in the morning. But when these are present, they are usually good indicators of how the arthritis is doing overall. A physician commonly asks about the severity of fatigue or how long the stiffness lasts in the morning to get an idea of how well the arthritis is being controlled.

Other Related Problems of Arthritis

In addition to joint pain and fatigue, other problems may come along with arthritis. *Fever* may be present and may be constant or may come and go. Since fever may be caused by many other medical problems, it is important to be sure that no other illnesses are present.

Some types of arthritis result in *loss of weight.* While some persons would view this a benefit, weight loss from arthritis is usually not welcome. This weight loss is due to the overall effect of the arthritis on the body and is often accompanied by loss of appetite. Since there are many causes of weight loss, it is important that other medical problems are evaluated and treated by your physician.

Many other signs can signal individual types of arthritis. For example, *rashes* on the skin are a frequent sign. Other changes in the skin can include *white or bluish discoloration of the fingers* when exposed to cold. *Unusual sensitivity to sunlight* with severe skin reactions may occur and some people experience *hair loss.*

Each of these problems may happen in more than one type of arthritis, and a few kinds of arthritis have certain typical combinations of feelings and signs. This often helps your physician in arriving at a proper diagnosis. Knowing the specific feelings and signs can help to improve treatment, since some treatments work well in certain kinds of arthritis and not in others. Table 2.1 shows some of the most common problems that may go along with arthritis of various types. These are discussed with the specific kinds of arthritis beginning on page 21.

Table 2.1
Some of the Most Common Types of Arthritis

Osteoarthritis Group	Inflammatory Arthritis Group
Osteoarthritis	Rheumatoid Arthritis
Bursitis	Gout (Gouty Arthritis)
Tendinitis	Systemic Lupus Erythematosus
Fibrositis (Fibromyalgia)	(Lupus or SLE)
	Polymyalgia Rheumatica
	Temporal Arteritis
	Ankylosing Spondylitis
	Juvenile Rheumatoid Arthritis
	Arthritis due to Infections
	Lyme Arthritis (Lyme Disease)
	"Staph" Arthritis
	Psoriatic Arthritis
	Scleroderma
	Vasculitis
	Sjogren's Syndrome

Arthritis Affects the Entire Body

Many forms of arthritis affect much more than the joints. Internal organs can be involved and may eventually cause the illness to be life-threatening. Fortunately, good treatment is available for most types of arthritis. The joint pain and other symptoms of the disease can be controlled.

Arthritis in the Foot

The foot is commonly affected by arthritis. Because the foot contains about one fourth of the body's bones and a large number of joints, arthritis can cause considerable foot pain and disability.

Some types of arthritis, such as gout, first affect the foot. Gout first attacks the large toe 75 percent of the time. When your foot hurts, you alter the way you walk and hold yourself. This can create stress and problems in other joints of the body such as the knees, hips, or back.

Seeking early care when there is discomfort in the foot can speed the diagnosis of the specific kind of arthritis, which can lead to earlier and more effective treatment. Try not to discount foot pain as foot fatigue or poorly fitting shoes until you are sure your problem is not more involved.

In osteoarthritis in the feet, the bones may become enlarged and the available motion of the joints may be decreased. These bone enlargements can cause increased pressure against the ground, the shoe, or a nearby bone. The body reacts by forming a corn or callus. This is especially common after age 40 or 50.

One common deformity in the foot is called "hammer toe." The toes move up over the top while the rounded bones in the front part of the foot protrude downward. The tendons pull the toes into the hammer-toe position (Figure 2.2). Another deformity may result when the larger joints in the middle of the foot change, destroying the arch of the foot.

These and other deformities change the shape of the foot. Pressure from shoes causes more callus and corn formation. Ready-made shoes are usually constructed for the "normal" shaped foot. Therefore, the foot with arthritis may need either a

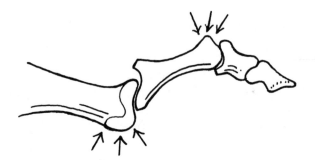

Figure 2.2. A diagram of *hammer toe.*

custom made shoe environment to avoid damage or surgery to change the deformity.

Over 100 Types

There are over 100 kinds of arthritis. Even experienced arthritis specialists may have trouble deciding which kind of arthritis is present in each case. To make it easier to understand, it helps to divide most kinds of arthritis into 2 groups, (Table 2.1).

Osteoarthritis

The first group of arthritis, osteoarthritis, is the most common and is related to the result of "wear-and-tear" changes in the joints, especially in the cartilage that covers the surface of the joints. The cartilage acts as a "cushion" for the forces put on the joint during activity.

Osteoarthritis occurs most commonly as the aging process occurs. It is most common in joints that hold up weight over the years or have been injured, such as the knees, hips, and spine. This is the kind of arthritis that many think of as "old age arthritis." Since this is the most well-known kind of arthritis, many people think that everyone who has arthritis is old. Most of us associate old age with arthritis because we remember a grandparent or other older person with swollen or painful joints such as the knees or the hands.

In fact, many older persons *do not* have arthritis, and many younger persons *do* have osteoarthritis. But it is also true that this "wear-and-tear" kind of arthritis is more common as we get older, usually after age 50. Another name for this kind of arthritis is *degenerative joint disease.*

Mary is a 51-year-old woman who enjoys golf. Over the past few years she noticed pain and stiffness in her knees. At first it was only occasional pain after unusual activity. Then the knee pain became constant and worsened when she played golf. She noticed no other joint pain or stiffness. She actually felt well except for the knee pain. She was not bothered by stiffness in the morning, but her knees hurt more and more during the day with activity. She asked if she should stop golf because of the pain.

She was found to have osteoarthritis in both knees. She began a regular program of exercise and medication and over a period of time had improvement in knee pain and stiffness. She has been able to continue playing golf with only occasional discomfort.

A few other kinds of arthritis and related diseases are also mainly a result of wear-and-tear changes around the joints and are managed much like osteoarthritis. These include many forms of *bursitis, tendinitis,* and other causes of inflammation in the tissues around the joints resulting in pain and stiffness. These problems are usually felt in *one* or only a few areas such as the shoulder or the hip. These are some of the most common causes of shoulder pain and are discussed on page 24.

Another very common problem is *fibrositis* (or fibromyalgia). This form of arthritis may cause severe pain and stiffness in many areas such as the back, the neck, the hips, and many other areas. This condition can be very disabling, but treatment is available. Fibrositis is discussed on page 25.

Inflammatory Types of Arthritis

The second group of types of arthritis includes those forms in which the linings of the joints become inflamed—inflammatory arthritis. In a few cases, the cause is known, but in most cases, the mystery remains. The joints become swollen and painful and may be warm or red. These kinds of arthritis may affect the hands, wrists, elbows, shoulders, knees, ankles, feet, neck, back, and hips and in any combination.

This type of arthritis is different from the first group of osteoarthritis-related arthritis in that there is often more than

This type of arthritis is different from the first group of osteoarthritis-related arthritis in that there is often more than joint pain to cause suffering. For example, there is frequently prominent stiffness upon rising in the morning. This stiffness may last hours or even all day, but often gradually wears off after 1 or 2 hours. This stiffness may return after you sit or rest for a few minutes during the day.

Another common problem with this type of arthritis is fatigue. There is usually a feeling of tiredness that can be as limiting as the joint pain. This fatigue may last all day and can severely limit a person's activity.

John and Susan on pages 2 and 11 are examples of inflammatory types of arthritis.

The exciting news is that as the arthritis improves, the bothersome stiffness in the morning and the tiredness usually improve, leaving the patient able to function. This is discussed later along with the specific types of arthritis.

There are a large number of types of arthritis that fit into this second grouping. However, these particular types usually share the problems of joint pain or stiffness, tiredness and fatigue, and stiffness upon rising in the morning. In addition, each specific kind of arthritis may have its own special problems such as rash, muscle weakness, kidney disease, or other internal organ illness.

How to Win with Arthritis

The goal of the person with arthritis is to change the disease from something disabling to something manageable. Winning with arthritis means that you become able to get around and do the activities you would like to do in reasonable comfort without side effects from medications.

CHAPTER THREE

Common Types of Arthritis

Let's look at a few of the most common types of arthritis. This will make it easier to understand the feelings you may have, what changes you might see, what tests might be suggested, and what the most effective treatment might be. The types of arthritis will be described in this chapter, and the treatment will be discussed in later chapters. We will not attempt to explain every type of arthritis in great detail, but there is a list of books and references on page 223 if you would like more extensive discussion of a specific form of arthritis. This book cannot replace proper diagnosis by your physician. Rather, the purpose of this book is to help you know that you can control and manage your arthritis. You can understand the facts about arthritis and manage your arthritis just as you manage other areas of your life.

Osteoarthritis

Osteoarthritis is the most common type of arthritis. It is more common in older persons, especially after age 50. It may happen earlier, especially if there was an earlier injury to a joint. For example, an athlete who injures a knee or an ankle may develop osteoarthritis in the injured joint.

21

Osteoarthritis is most common in joints that are required to bear weight over the years such as the knees, hips, and spine. It usually comes on gradually over months or years. Except for the pain in the affected joint, the person usually feels well. There is no unusual tiredness or fatigue. If there is stiffness upon rising in the morning, it is usually mild and goes away in a few minutes. No internal organs are affected by osteoarthritis.

Another form of osteoarthritis may affect the hands or other joints even though they have not had excessive wear over the years. This is most common in women and may affect women even in their 30s. This disease may be inherited, occurring in other female family members as well. This form of osteoarthritis can be severe enough to mimic other more serious forms of arthritis such as rheumatoid arthritis but does not usually have as severe a pattern. Often this form of arthritis affects only the hands—it does not strike many other joints as the more serious types of arthritis commonly do.

The joints affected by osteoarthritis may be painful and swollen. The joints may be warm to the touch. There may be difficulty in using the joint for activities such as walking when the knee or hip are affected. Or, if the hands are affected there may be trouble opening jars, using buttons, or with other tasks.

In the hands, the joints most typically affected are the joints in the fingers nearest the fingernails and the joint at the base of the thumb. (See Figure 3.1.) In osteoarthritis, when the joint is at rest, there is often little or no pain but after the arthritis has been present for a number of years the pain may become constant. When the joint is moved, there is often a grating or crackling feeling (which is called *crepitus*).

Other joints may also be affected by osteoarthritis. The feet, the neck, and the middle and lower part of the back may also be attacked. The shoulders and ankles may also be involved, but usually less often than the knees or hips.

X-rays show changes in the joints that are usually easy to detect in osteoarthritis as the cartilage space is narrowed. (See Figure 3.2.) There are often definite changes present in the joints as seen by x-ray by the time a person has enough pain to seek medical help. This may not be true in other kinds of arthritis. A

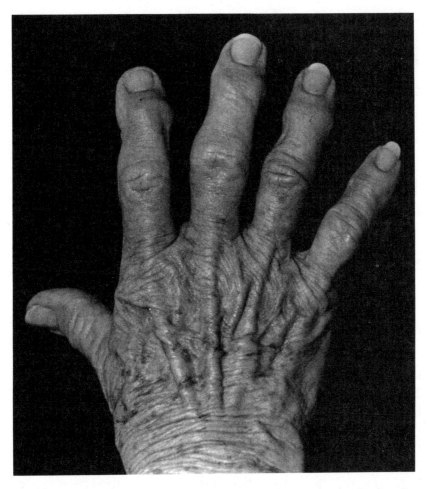

Figure 3.1.   Osteoarthritis often affects the joints nearest the fingernails.

few other tests may help eliminate other causes of arthritis. Examining a sample of joint fluid may confirm the diagnosis of osteoarthritis. Different kinds of arthritis may cause different changes in the joint fluid. This test can be done by your physician in his office with very little discomfort. Blood tests are helpful to be sure no other problems are present.

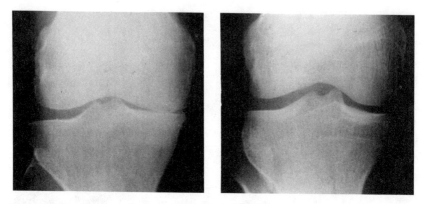

Figure 3.2.   X-rays of osteoarthritis in a knee (left) and a normal knee (right).

Bursitis and Tendinitis

Bursitis causes pain around a joint that can be very severe and limiting. A bursa is an area or sac through which tendons and muscles move smoothly. When bursitis is present, there is pain on any movement of the muscles or tendons.

The first sensation of bursitis may be pain near a joint that worsens when the joint is moved or with pressure on the joint. The pain may be mild or very severe and may last from a few days to months or even years. The areas most commonly affected are shoulders and hips. Other areas that may develop bursitis are knees, elbows, and buttocks. At times, certain repetitive movements of an arm in one direction or in one activity (such as hammering) may trigger an attack of bursitis, especially if the activity has not been done recently.

Bursitis can be painful and incapacitating. It can accompany arthritis and can make the actual source of pain difficult to distinguish.

There is pain with pressure in the area of the bursa, and swelling and warmth may be present as well. The pain is often most severe with pressure on the front or side of the shoulder or at the side of the hip. Other areas that may be affected are the front of the knees (housemaid's knees), the buttocks (weaver's bottom), and around the elbows.

The most common causes of bursitis are wear-and-tear changes in the tissues that make up the bursa. Although bursitis is not true osteoarthritis, we discuss it here since it can cause similar feelings, and the treatment is similar in many ways. There are other causes of bursitis such as infection and gout. Your physician will want to eliminate these causes since they need other specific treatment.

If the pain is severe, you should see your physician. Other more serious conditions must be eliminated. X-rays and blood tests may be taken to help guide treatment.

Tendinitis refers to inflammation of a tendon that attaches a muscle to a bone. The inflammation may cause pain, swelling, warmth, and difficulty using the nearby joint. "Tennis elbow," for example, is tendinitis of the muscles that attach at the elbow. It is common in persons who repeatedly make the movements that are done in tennis, as well as baseball, golf, and other activities. Other areas that may be bothered by tendinitis are the shoulder and the Achilles tendon near the heel. Tendinitis may cause severe pain with use of the muscle or nearby joint.

Tendinitis, like bursitis, is most often caused by overuse or wear-and-tear changes in the tissues that make up the tendon. Although not a true arthritis, it commonly is found along with arthritis and may be difficult to distinguish as a cause of pain around a joint.

Fibrositis (Fibromyalgia)

Fibrositis (fibromyalgia) is a common cause of pain in the muscles and joints of the arms, legs, neck, and back. It is one of the most common causes of pain and stiffness. It is most common in females. Five times as many females are affected as males. The cause is unknown, although some cases have begun following an injury that may be quite mild. Some cases seem to be linked to stress or emotion. Some researchers feel there may be a viral cause. The term *fibrositis* implies that there is inflammation of fibrous tissue in the muscles and other tissues, but this has not been proven when samples of those tissues were studied. This disorder goes by other names including fibromyositis and tension myalgia.

Since fibrositis can at times cause signs and feelings similar to osteoarthritis, bursitis, and tendinitis, it is included in this group of arthritis and related disorders.

Most persons with fibrositis feel widespread aching in their muscles and joints. The areas most commonly affected are the neck, shoulders, elbows, knees, and back (Figure 3.3). Although there may be difficulty doing daily work or caring for the home, most persons can complete these duties despite not feeling well. The symptoms and feelings usually come and go and commonly are associated with severe fatigue, headache, and depression. Most persons have difficulty sleeping.

They may be unable to go to sleep or may not feel rested when they awaken in the morning. On arising, they may feel stiffness in the muscles and joints.

The feelings of pain and stiffness in fibrositis are very widespread, unlike the usual bursitis or tendinitis that is local- ized to a single area. In fact, if there are not many areas involved, then it does not fit the typical picture of fibrositis.

With fibrositis, there is no joint swelling, no loss of move- ment of the joints, and no true muscle weakness. Usually the only abnormal findings are tender areas over the neck, shoulder blades, lower back, elbows, and knees. These tender areas are called *trigger areas*. In fact, if a joint is warm or swollen or does not move properly then there is probably another problem present.

Fibrositis can occur with or without the presence of another problem such as rheumatoid arthritis, systemic lupus erythe- matosus (SLE or Lupus), polymyalgia rheumatica, or other inter- nal organ diseases.

The diagnosis is difficult at times because there are no specific laboratory tests and no abnormal x-ray findings in fi- brositis. There may be a need to have more than one examination to be sure no other disorders are being overlooked.

Inflammatory Types of Arthritis

The second large group of types of arthritis includes those in which the linings of the joints become inflamed, causing pain,

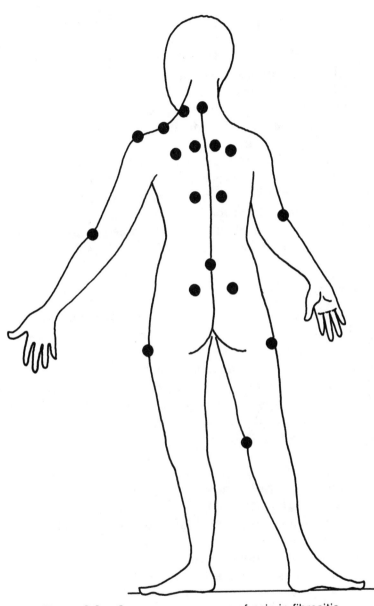

Figure 3.3. Some common areas of pain in fibrositis.

swelling, and often warmth and redness in and around the joints. The causes of most of these types of arthritis are not known. Almost every joint may be attacked, including the hands, wrists, elbows, shoulders, hips, knees, ankles, feet, neck, back, and jaws.

These types of arthritis are often more limiting than the first type—osteoarthritis. These disorders may also cause more severe deformity and permanent changes in the joints. They are also more likely to result in crippling. Severe fatigue is common and may be the most limiting symptom. Stiffness in the morning is often severe, lasting hours or most of the day. These types of arthritis are more likely to have internal organ involvement. Medications are available that can slow down or halt the progress of the disease, but they may have some unwanted side effects, and therefore must be used with a physician's direction.

Rheumatoid Arthritis

The most common type of arthritis in this group is rheumatoid arthritis. This attacks over 10 million Americans. The cause of rheumatoid arthritis is not known, but it is more common in women than men and can occur at almost any age. It usually comes on gradually with pain, stiffness, and swelling in the hands, wrists, elbows, shoulders, knees, ankles, or feet. There is usually bothersome stiffness in all the joints upon rising in the morning. Fatigue is usually very prominent. In fact, most people complain about fatigue as much or more than the actual joint pain. Fever, weight loss, and other symptoms may be present. Rheumatoid arthritis can cause so many different problems that it may be confused with many other diseases.

The joints may be painful, swollen, and warm to touch. Muscles may become smaller and weaker. The pain and stiffness cause difficulty performing daily activities at work and at home. It may become difficult to dress or to use a knife or fork. In severe cases, walking as well as most other activities needed for daily living may be severely limited.

In rheumatoid arthritis, some blood tests and x-rays can be helpful in making a diagnosis and in planning treatment. In most cases, there are findings in talking with the patient and on examination that will allow a tentative diagnosis. The blood test that is widely used to help in the diagnosis determines the *rheumatoid factor*. This factor is present in 70 to 80 percent of patients with rheumatoid arthritis. The rheumatoid factor may also be present in diseases other than rheumatoid arthritis. Other blood tests are helpful to evaluate for problems such as anemia that can contribute to the fatigue. Your physician can guide you.

X-rays are often taken to check for changes that may occur in rheumatoid arthritis (Figure 3.4). X-rays of hands, wrists, and feet are usually the most helpful for detecting early changes due to rheumatoid arthritis. Other joints may show these changes later, depending on how affected each joint happens to be.

If x-rays show subtle changes in the joints called *erosions*, then this may be a sign that a more serious arthritis may be present—one that has the potential for destructive changes. Since this is a very early finding, it allows for planning the most effective treatment available to slow down or stop the progress of the disease. It provides an opportunity to prevent deformity and loss of use of the joints with the most effective treatment as early as possible. This can be done long before there are any other outwardly visible signs of deformity or crippling.

Treatment of rheumatoid arthritis (discussed in Chapter 4) is aimed at control of the pain and maintaining use of the joints. It takes time, but in the majority of patients the pain can be very adequately controlled. The goal should be to have enough control so that the person affected is able to be comfortable and to do the desired daily activities.

Five percent or less of rheumatoid arthritis patients have severe crippling. With proper treatment, most patients can now view rheumatoid arthritis as being inconvenient but not terrible or devastating. Most persons can continue to do most of the activities they choose with some modifications at times.

The best control of rheumatoid arthritis may be gained within the first year or two of the onset of the disease. Therefore, to have a better chance at control of the arthritis try to have the earliest and most effective treatment possible.

Gout (Gouty Arthritis)

Gout is a form of arthritis that often hits suddenly with very severe pain. The pain usually becomes more severe over a few hours. The large toe is the most commonly affected joint and

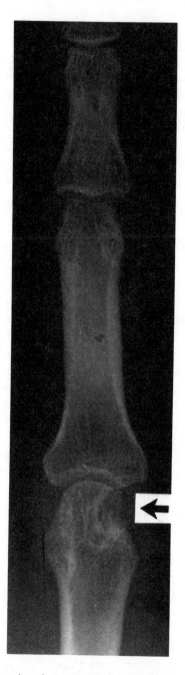

Figure 3.4. An example of destruction of bone in a finger joint with rheumatoid arthritis.

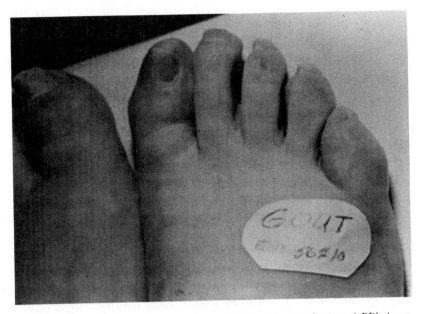

Figure 3.5. An example of acute gout attack in the first and fifth toes. (Photograph courtesy of the American Podiatric Medical Association.)

is the first joint attacked in 75 percent of cases. The toe is painful, swollen, and often warm and red. The pain usually makes it hard to stand or walk. The pain may be so severe that even the weight of bedsheets causes severe discomfort.

Other joints commonly involved are the ankle, knee, wrist, and elbow. Most often, one joint is attacked alone, but it may also happen in several joints at the same time. This may become more common if gout goes untreated over a long period of time. If left untreated, gout can cause a severe arthritis with deformity (Figure 3.5).

An attack of gout may happen after an illness or surgery, after excess alcohol intake, with some medications, and with other medical problems. It is much more common in men (usually over 40-years-old) than in women. Kidney stones may also occur in persons who have gout.

The cause of gout is a high uric acid level in the blood. Uric acid is normally present in the blood as a product of the body's use of protein. If the body produces too much uric acid or if the kidneys do not remove enough uric acid from the blood, the level of uric acid may increase. If the level remains high for a period of time, uric acid may become concentrated around joints or in the kidneys. This may result in an attack of arthritis or a kidney stone.

Diagnosis of gouty arthritis is most accurately made by examining a sample of fluid obtained from the joint. Under a special microscope, crystals of uric acid can be seen that confirm gout. A blood test is taken to measure the level of uric acid, which is usually high. A high blood uric acid level makes a person more likely to develop gout but alone does not make the diagnosis definite.

Systemic Lupus Erythematosus (SLE or Lupus)

Systemic lupus erythematosus, also called SLE or lupus, is another inflammatory arthritis that is most common in women, especially in the ages 20 to 40. It may also occur in children as well as older men and women and is more common in African-American women.

The cause of systemic lupus erythematosus is not known. There is inflammation in the blood vessels that can result in disease in almost any organ. The most common problem is arthritis. There may be pain and swelling in the hands, wrists, elbows, shoulders, knees, ankles, and feet. There may be pain and stiffness in the neck, back, jaws, and hips. There may be severe fatigue and stiffness in the joints upon arising in the morning. The arthritis may appear much like rheumatoid arthritis, especially early in the disease.

Many other problems can happen with lupus. There is almost always fatigue, and there may be fever and rash. Up to forty percent of patients have a rash across the cheeks that has been called the *"butterfly rash."* Twenty percent or more may become *unusually sensitive to sunlight* with the appearance of a rash and fever. The fingers and toes may become *unusually sensitive to cool temperatures* so that they turn white or blue when exposed to cold. *Hair loss* may be a problem. About 50 percent of persons with lupus develop kidney disease that can lead to kidney failure. Other internal organs can be affected including the brain, the heart, the lungs, and the liver. Blood disorders can cause anemia, bleeding, infecticn, and blood clots.

Lupus can be very difficult to diagnose because it can mimic many other diseases. This delay in diagnosis may add to the frustration these persons feel from the disease alone.

Blood tests are helpful in making the diagnosis of lupus. About 95 percent of persons with lupus have a positive blood test for antinuclear antibody (ANA). Other blood tests are also helpful. Although at times difficult, the overall pattern and combination of problems usually allows proper diagnosis.

Polymyalgia Rheumatica

Polymyalgia rheumatica is a strange-sounding disease that affects persons over 50 (and usually over 60). The cause is unknown. Polymyalgia rheumatica often occurs in a person who has been quite healthy otherwise. There is a sudden or gradual onset of severe pain and stiffness in the muscles around the shoulders and upper arms and in the hips and thighs. Usually there is no swelling in the joints, but there is severe fatigue and severe stiffness on arising in the morning. The pain is often so severe that it is hard to turn over in bed at night! There may be mild fever, weight loss, and poor appetite.

There is little visual evidence of the disease but it causes great discomfort. There is usually prominent tenderness in the muscles of the upper arms, shoulders, and over the thighs and hips.

Testing including blood tests is usually done to look for other diseases. The most useful test is the blood sedimentation rate. The results are abnormally high in polymyalgia rheumatica. It is important to look for other medical problems that may mimic this disease. Especially important is a disease that can exist along WITH polymyalgia rheumatica called temporal arteritis. This is discussed next.

Temporal Arteritis

Temporal arteritis is a disease caused by inflammation in the arteries and takes its name from problems in the temporal arteries on the side of the head just in front of the ear. This disease affects mainly those persons over 50 (often over 60). Headache is most common and usually prominent. There may be pain in the muscles of the jaws when chewing food. There may also be fever, weight loss, and fatigue. There may be pain and stiffness in the shoulders, upper arms and in the thighs and hips just as in polymyalgia rheumatica. If untreated, there may be sudden loss of vision in an eye or other severe complications. This is because the arteries involved become narrowed and may stop the blood flow to part of the eye or part of the brain.

There may be tenderness on touching the temple area at the sides of the head. There may be tenderness over the upper arms, shoulders and thighs. There may be little else to see.

Blood tests show a very high sedimentation rate, just as in polymyalgia rheumatica. In fact, both diseases may be present at the same time. A sample biopsy of a temporal artery under local anesthesia may provide the diagnosis. This is usually done on an outpatient basis.

Ankylosing Spondylitis

In ankylosing spondylitis, the joints of the lower back—the sacroiliac joints and lumbar spine—become inflamed. This problem strikes men more commonly than women and begins most typically in young men from teen years to age 30. It often starts as pain in the lower back that may come and go and is often thought to be from a strain or injury. However, the pain stays and gradually worsens.

There is usually stiffness in the lower back on arising in the morning that lasts a few minutes to several hours. Fatigue is often present but is usually not as severe as in rheumatoid arthritis. In this disease, prolonged inactivity usually causes more pain and stiffness, while in lower back injuries rest usually reduces the pain.

There may be pain and stiffness in other areas, such as the shoulders, hips, and other joints. About half of the people with this disease have arthritis in the shoulders or hips.

After a few years, there may be pain in the middle part of the back (the thoracic spine). After 5 to 10 years, there may be pain and stiffness in the neck as well. There may be a gradual stiffening of the spine so that movement of the lower and middle back and the neck may be more difficult. Stiffness in the back may limit bending and stooping over. Neck stiffness is often noticed when there is difficulty turning the head while driving.

There may be few signs visible of this arthritis at first. Difficulty moving the back, shoulders or hips may be noticed. On examination, your physician can detect more subtle changes that show the problems of movement in the spine.

Other problems that may occur in ankylosing spondylitis include inflammation of part of the eye called *iritis*. This requires diagnosis and proper treatment by an opthalmologist to avoid loss of vision. This disease may also attack the lungs, heart valves, and can cause pressure on nerves as they leave the spinal cord and pass through the bones of the spine.

The cause of ankylosing spondylitis is not known. However, over 90 percent of persons with this arthritis have a positive blood test that marks their higher tendency toward developing ankylosing spondylitis. This marker is called the HLA-B27 antigen and is inherited from a parent. It is thought that those with this tendency may come into contact with something in their environment that "triggers" the arthritis to begin. This might be a virus, bacteria, or other unknown contact in our daily lives. Research will probably give us a good idea of the nature of this trigger in the future.

Diagnosis of ankylosing spondylitis is usually made after discussion and examination along with x-rays of the back. Blood tests for HLA-B27 antigen may be helpful. Proper treatment is especially important and very effective in prevention of deformity of the spine.

Juvenile Rheumatoid Arthritis

As we discussed previously, arthritis can attack almost any age, including children. A type of arthritis that looks similar to rheumatoid arthritis (but begins before age 16) is called juvenile rheumatoid arthritis. This actually has several different forms. It may start as an illness with fever and rash with very little joint pain and swelling. This form may cause heart disease in some children.

Another form may affect only one or a few joints, most commonly the knee. It may cause inflammation of a portion of the eye (iritis) and if not treated properly can cause loss of vision.

Yet another form may affect many joints and behaves more like the adult type of rheumatoid arthritis. This may continue for years with joint pain, swelling, and loss of use of the joints if not treated.

The cause of these forms of arthritis is not known, just as the cause is not known in adults. The outlook is better in children since 50 percent or more of children with these types of arthritis may improve and in many cases the signs of the arthritis may disappear.

Arthritis Due to Infections

Some types of arthritis can be caused by certain infections. These are important to discover since there is effective treatment with antibiotics and the arthritis may become more severe if not treated properly.

Lyme Arthritis (Lyme Disease)

Lyme Arthritis is the most recent type of arthritis for which the cause has been discovered. Fifteen years ago, researchers from Yale University described several patients in the Lyme River area with what came to be known as Lyme disease. This condition has now been found in many states, most commonly in Connecticut, Massachusetts, New York, New Jersey, Wisconsin, Minnesota, California, Oregon, and Washington. Some researchers believe that Lyme disease may be a recent European import since it resembles disorders described there over 100 years ago.

Lyme disease is caused by an infection due to an organism called Borrelia burgdorferi. It is carried by field mice and deer who pass it to the ticks that live on their bodies. The tick then bites a human and passes the infection. Some researchers believe that other insects might also transmit the infection. Lyme disease is most common in the spring and summer months.

The 3 Stages of Lyme Disease

Stage 1 occurs days to months after the tick bite. A rash (called erythema chronicum migrans) may begin as a single spot in the groin or other area and gradually become larger. Other areas of rash may be present. There may be flu-like feelings with fever, joint and muscle pain, headache, chills, sore throat, and stiff neck. Many people do not remember having a tick bite or rash. Blood tests for Lyme disease at this time may be negative.

About 10 percent of people with this disease progress to stage 2. Headaches and weakness are common feelings due to nerve involvement. Facial weakness (Bell's Palsy) can occur. Heart disease occurs in about 10 percent of the people and may cause irregular heart beats or heart failure. Death is rare, but heart disease is the most common cause. A blood test might still be negative in this stage.

Stage 3 is hallmarked by arthritis and may follow the tick bite by several years. About 10 percent of the people get chronic arthritis with pain, stiffness, and swelling in the joints that may look like rheumatoid arthritis. The blood test for Lyme disease is usually positive in this stage. Many persons who live in areas where the disease is common may have positive blood tests but not actually have the disease. Symptoms and illnesses should not be blamed on Lyme disease without proper confirmation.

Treatment is with antibiotics, which are given as early as possible. Sometimes antibiotics are given if there is a high suspicion of Lyme disease even if the blood tests are not positive. Antibiotics used in stage 1 include tetracycline or penicillin. With severe disease such as heart involvement or arthritis, high doses of penicillin or other antibiotics are recommended.

"Staph" Arthritis

A severe type of arthritis is caused by the staphylococcus bacteria, which is commonly found on our skin. If this bacteria attacks a joint, it can cause severe joint damage in a few days if not treated. This infection usually attacks only one joint and may appear after an injury or skin infection near the joint. The joint (especially the knee, wrist, or ankle) becomes very painful and may have warmth, swelling, and redness. Movement and use of the joint are difficult.

"Staph" arthritis requires immediate treatment with antibiotics and may need surgery in some cases. This type of arthritis may occur in a person already affected with arthritis, such as rheumatoid arthritis. If a single joint becomes very painful or swollen then evaluation by a physician is needed as soon as possible.

Other infections can cause arthritis, including gonorrhea, a sexually transmitted disease, and the AIDS virus, Human Immunodeficiency Virus (HIV). The references on page 223 give suggestions for more detailed discussion of these and other less common infections that can cause arthritis.

Psoriatic Arthritis

Psoriasis causes a rash on the skin, often with red, scaly patches over the elbow, hands, knees, and other areas. This is usually long lasting and can often be controlled with medication used on the skin or by other treatment. Your physician can make the diagnosis and plan treatment.

Some persons with psoriasis develop a disorder that may resemble rheumatoid arthritis. It may affect the hands, wrists, elbows, shoulders, knees, ankles, feet, and spine. Most often the hands, feet, and a few other joints are attacked. There is often stiffness in the morning upon arising and fatigue just as in rheumatoid arthritis. The arthritis may happen with or without worsening of the skin rash of psoriasis. Treatment is discussed in Chapter 4.

Scleroderma

Scleroderma means "hard skin," which is what happens to the skin of persons who have this disease. It can vary from a small area of skin in children to a form that affects the skin and internal organs and is life-threatening in adults.

The cause of scleroderma is not known. There is overproduction of collagen, a building block for skin and other structures in the body. It begins to replace other normal tissues in the body, so that those organs affected do not work normally. Also, blood supply to these organs is often decreased.

An early feeling in scleroderma is discoloration of the fingers on cold exposure which can be painful (Raynaud's phenomenon). Later, the skin can become thickened and hard so that body structures are frozen in one position. The skin may break and ulcers form. Fingers may lose their blood supply. If internal organs such as the lungs or kidney are affected it can be life-threatening. There are also milder forms of the disease with less internal organ involvement.

There is no prevention or cure for scleroderma at this time. Treatment is directed at the above symptoms. The disease may "level out" and progress no further at some point. Research is still being done to find the cause and better treatment for this disease.

Vasculitis

In vasculitis the blood vessels (especially arteries) are damaged, usually by abnormal proteins circulating in the blood. As the blood vessels are damaged, some organs lose their oxygen and nutrient supply and no longer work properly. There are many different causes of vasculitis, most of which are not very well understood. In many cases, the body's immune system starts to damage blood vessels in the same way that it attacks foreign invaders of the body.

The disease affects all ages and may involve only the skin or may affect internal organs and be fatal. Rash is common, as is joint pain and stiffness. The fingers may turn white on cold exposure as in scleroderma. There may be gangrene in the fingers and toes from loss of blood supply. The kidneys, lungs, and heart may be involved. Proper diagnosis and treatment is needed as early as possible to prevent more serious and irreversible organ damage.

Diagnosis is usually made by biopsy of an organ or x-ray of the arteries. Treatment is most commonly high doses of a cortisone derivative. Other medications may be needed to control the disease. With newer treatments and medications, the survival rate in vasculitis has improved dramatically. Vasculitis requires specialized and individual treatment with close monitoring by your physician.

Sjogren's Syndrome

Sjogren's syndrome is actually most commonly seen along with other problems, especially rheumatoid arthritis. Sjogren's syndrome results in dryness of the eyes and mouth because the glands in these areas do not give the normal amount or quality of tears or saliva.

The cause of Sjogren's syndrome is not known. It is most common in women, and 50 percent or more of persons affected have rheumatoid arthritis or other types of arthritis. There is often swelling of the parotid glands on the sides of the face (the same glands affected by mumps). Other internal organ diseases and blood abnormalities can occur as well.

Two Kinds of Arthritis?

It is possible to have more than one kind of arthritis. Having one type does not prevent the development of another. For example, osteoarthritis often develops in a person who has rheumatoid arthritis for a number of years. The rheumatoid arthritis may cause more rapid wearing away of the joint cartilage so that osteoarthritis develops.

In some women, osteoarthritis occurs in the fingers, and often has happened to other females in the family. Some of these persons are unlucky enough to later develop rheumatoid arthritis in addition to the previous osteoarthritis. The rheumatoid arthritis is treated as it would usually be treated.

Another common combination is arthritis caused by infection and rheumatoid or other arthritis. Some patients with arthritis seem to have a higher risk for infection. At times, the medications used for treatment may also raise the risk of infection.

One combination of arthritis that happens only rarely is rheumatoid arthritis and gout in the same person. The reason for this rare occurrence together is not known.

When arthritis seems to "change course" or become more severe, then it is possible that a second type of arthritis has developed. When only one out of many joints becomes worse, then infection as a new cause of arthritis is considered. It is also possible that the previous arthritis has simply worsened. Your physician can help to make the correct decision in these situations.

In the next chapter, we will discuss the basic treatment for arthritis in general and some specific treatments for the more common types of arthritis.

CHAPTER FOUR

A Basic Treatment Plan

Anyone with arthritis can begin to control the disease by using a *basic treatment plan*. This plan outlines the steps you can take each day to manage the pain and stiffness and prevent arthritis from limiting your activities. This basic plan is an effective beginning. Then by adding specific measures for your own situation with the help of your physician, you can be sure that you are doing all you can to win with your arthritis.

Heat and Exercises Are Important

Heat and exercises are a basic part of the treatment in almost every type of arthritis. With the use of heat, the stiff joints and muscles loosen. Using heat in combination with exercises allows easier movement of the joints and helps reduce the pain, swelling, and stiffness. At first, when there is much stiffness and pain, the heat will make it easier to start the exercises.

We suggest the use of *moist heat* twice daily such as a shower, bathtub, warm towels, or pool. Use the moist heat for 10 to 15 minutes each morning and evening. A heated pool or whirlpool is the ideal way to give heat to the joints. A pool is often used with hospital patients for very severe attacks of arthritis to allow exercises to begin. If you do not have access to a pool, a warm shower or bathtub is also very effective.

43

Many people have difficulty getting in and out of a bathtub because of the pain and stiffness. In these cases, a shower is preferred using a stool or chair with rubber tips on the legs for safety. Most people actually find the shower to be the quickest and easiest form of moist heat for regular use. (See Figure 4.1.)

Warm towels or hot packs (called hydrocollator packs) are effective. Hydrocollator packs can be obtained through a medical supply store or your physician. Both of these methods require effort in preparing the towels or packs which may be harder for people with severe arthritis. Moist heating pads are easier to use but may not be as effective. Avoid those pads that create too much heat. The heat should not be uncomfortable. Your physician can guide you to specific brands of heat pads available to best fit your own situation.

A dry heating pad is easier to use, although one of the forms of moist heat is usually more effective, especially when the pain and stiffness are more severe. The important thing is the effect—that is, improvement in pain so that exercises can be done more easily. Dry heat may do well enough once there has been improvement in the arthritis.

Another excellent form of heat when arthritis involves the hands or feet is the use of a heated mixture of paraffin and mineral oil. This is an old treatment, and must be done correctly to be safe. A small and convenient device is available that can be used at home with little trouble. For many persons, it makes a major difference in their flexibility and comfort when used regularly. Have your physician or physical therapist show you the paraffin/oil treatment and decide if this works better for you than warm water or bath.

Heated pool
Warm shower
Whirlpool
Warm bathtub
Warm, moist towels
Hydrocollator packs
Moist heating pads
Paraffin–mineral oil therapeutic mixture

Figure 4.1. Common forms of moist heat

The form of heat that works best and is the easiest for you should be continued. When the pain is gone, then the heat can be used only when needed rather than twice daily.

Ice may give relief when applied to an inflamed joint for 10 to 15 minutes several times each day. Ice is often most helpful when arthritis is acute or severe. Ice can be put in a plastic bag and the bag applied to the joint, or a standard ice bag may be used. The ice should not be put directly on the skin. If ice gives more relief than heat, it can be continued. Some persons find the best relief when ice treatments are alternated with moist heat treatments. However, most arthritis patients find moist heat to be more effective. Choose the form of heat or the combination of heat and ice that works best for you.

Exercises Are Important

Exercises are important in most types of arthritis. These special exercises may be the most important part of a treatment program for many persons. Exercises in arthritis accomplish two important goals. (See Figure 4.2.)

Muscles around joints affected by arthritis often become smaller and weaker. This gives less support to the very joints that need more than usual support. Exercises increase the strength of muscles gradually over a period of weeks to months. However, exercises are one of the most important parts of treatment over the long term.

Exercises keep the joints mobile and muscles stronger so that activity and usual daily functions can be continued. We spend a lot of time in our clinic teaching the importance of exercises. We find that persons who are able to do their exercises regularly are much more likely to improve and remain active and pain-free. People who cannot do exercises often see less improvement in their pain control and mobility.

Improves flexibility of joints = Makes joints more limber
Increases strength of muscles = Gives support to arthritic joints

Figure 4.2.   Benefits of exercise in arthritis

In many cases, if only one part of the treatment could be accomplished we would want it to be the exercises. We are often told by patients that it is the exercises that make a major difference in their improvement. They tell us that when they exercise they improve, and when they don't exercise regularly their arthritis worsens.

The *specific exercises* for each joint are discussed in Chapter 5. It is best to strengthen all of the muscles that support a joint attacked by arthritis. For example, it is helpful to strengthen the muscles of the hip and the back to improve support for the knee.

It usually requires weeks to learn the exercises effectively and to be able to perform the correct number of repetitions twice daily. A commitment on your part to follow through with the program is a must.

You may need to begin with only one repetition of the first exercise. You should have no more pain after you finish than when you begin exercising. If you experience severe pain while exercising, you should stop. Then at the next session try one or two repetitions. When you have mastered this number, try three or four repetitions, gradually increasing the number of exercises and repetitions. The goal is to perform 10 to 20 of each exercise twice daily. This is the level which seems to work well in most patients to maintain the highest level of strength and flexibility.

There will be some days when you are uncomfortable or tired and would rather not exercise. You must overcome your reluctance and begin a regular program of twice daily exercises to be done *every* day—good days and bad days as well. When your arthritis improves, don't stop the regular exercise program. It can be adjusted for more convenience, but should be continued indefinitely.

The use of moist heat along with the exercises makes them easier and less painful. For example, exercises can be done in the warm shower or pool. Once you are able to tolerate a regular program, these exercises will be more effective in producing flexible joints and stronger muscles.

If your arthritis is severe or if you are not used to exercises, start slowly but don't allow yourself to avoid the moist heat and exercises. Remember, there is also no limit on exercises by age! It may be necessary to begin your heat and exercise program with the help of regular visits to a physical therapist. Then as you improve you can manage the program at home with visits to the therapist when needed.

Rest Is a Vital Part of Treatment

Rest is also important in arthritis. When a joint is swollen and inflamed, it does not usually help to continue to try to use it normally. It is even possible that the underlying arthritis may advance if an inflamed joint such as the knee has continued use and weight bearing. Rest can be given to a single joint until the pain improves, or if many joints are involved it may even require bedrest for brief periods.

Rest periods can be very helpful during the day. Periods of rest by lying down or reclining for 15 to 30 minutes late in the morning and late in the afternoon can greatly help the pain and may make the rest of the day easier. Some office workers relax behind their desk and continue to work. It is not necessary to sleep or to be totally inactive. As the pain and swelling improve, the rest periods become less necessary and can be shortened or stopped.

In some types of arthritis, especially those in the inflammatory group, rest is important to help the fatigue. When the fatigue is great during periods of more active arthritis, the rest periods late in the morning and late in the afternoon will allow the rest of the day and evening to be of better quality. Also, proper rest at night is needed. It may at times be necessary to allow up to 10 hours of bedrest at night to help fatigue.

You will find it very helpful to *pace yourself with daily activities.* Try to break your work into periods with a few minutes rest in between. For example, mowing the lawn or cleaning could be done in 2 or 3 sessions with a few minutes break for coffee or rest. This may sound as if it would lower your work and productivity, but the overall amount of work accomplished will probably be equal or greater. And at the end, you are much more likely to have energy reserved for other activities.

There are some activities such as a long day of shopping, recreation activities, or traveling that may cause more severe fatigue. It is a good idea to try to rest as much as possible *before* the activity. Then be prepared to take the necessary time to recover from the activity.

The more bothersome the fatigue, the more important proper rest periods and rest at night will become. When the arthritis improves, then you can gradually lessen the number of rest periods. Families often notice improvement in a person's energy and overall activity level when proper rest is allowed.

Medications for Treatment

Along with moist heat, exercises, and proper rest, *medications* may greatly improve the pain, stiffness, and swelling in arthritis. There are a number of different types of medications that can be helpful. The *anti-inflammatory drugs* are the most commonly used group of medications for most types of arthritis. There are two types commonly used, the *cortisone derivatives* and the *noncortisone* or *nonsteroid anti-inflammatory drugs* (*NSAIDS*).

Cortisone Derivatives

The strongest anti-inflammatory drugs are the *cortisone derivatives*. These are a group of medications which control inflammation very effectively. Table 4.1 gives a few of the most commonly used cortisone derivatives. These are effective, but they have some side effects. Therefore, they must be used carefully and under medical supervision. If given in high enough doses, these medications can control the pain and swelling in

Table 4.1
Anti-Inflammatory Drugs—Cortisone Derivatives

Trade Name	Generic Name
Deltasone, Metacortin	Prednisone
Orasone	None
Medrol	Methylprednisolone
Aristocort	Triamcinolone
Decadron, Hexadrol	Dexamethasone

most cases of arthritis. However, they bring along some serious side effects, especially if used in high doses or over a long time. (See Table 4.2.)

To avoid the side effects of the cortisone derivatives, they are sometimes given by local injection into a joint. This can usually be done with little or no risk of side effects. In most cases there is improvement in pain and stiffness in the single joint within a few days. The improvement may last 6 weeks or more. The injection may be repeated, usually at intervals of no sooner than a few months, although each person is different. In about 15 percent of the cases, there may not be a very good or long-lasting improvement after an injection. This is especially true in those cases of osteoarthritis that have been present for many years so that there is little remaining active inflammation.

Table 4.2
Some of the Most Common Possible
Side Effects of Cortisone Derivatives*

Weight gain
Fluid retention (edema)
Hypertension (high blood pressure)
Gastric irritation and bleeding
Possible peptic ulcer disease and other intestinal problems
Osteoporosis (bone thinning)
Thin and more fragile skin, easy bruising
Acne
Delayed healing of cuts and wounds
Certain types of cataracts
Glaucoma
Increased chance of infection
Higher blood glucose (can aggravate diabetes mellitus)
Can suppress normal cortisone production
Menstrual irregularities
Other muscle and bone problems
Depression and other mental health disorders
Increased body hair growth
Changes in blood triglycerides

*Side effects often depend on the size of the dose and the length of treatment with the medication

Noncortisone Anti-Inflammatory Drugs

The second major type of anti-inflammatory medications used include the noncortisone anti-inflammatory drugs (also called the nonsteroid anti-inflammatory drugs or NSAIDs). (See Table 4.3.) These medications attempt to give the benefits of the cortisone derivatives in arthritis without the side effects. However, they are less potent, and they do have their own set of possible side effects. The majority of people with arthritis find one of this group of drugs that gives good relief of joint pain and swelling with no serious side effects. (See Table 4.4.)

Table 4.3
Some Common Noncortisone Anti-Inflammatory Drugs*

Trade Name	Generic Name
Advil	Ibuprofen
Anaprox	Naproxyn
Ansaid	Flurbiprofen
(See Table 4.5)	Aspirin products
Clinoril	Sulindac
Disalcid	Salsalate
Dolobid	Diflunisal
Feldene	Piroxicam
Indocin	Indomethacin
Meclomen	Meclofenamate
Medipren	Ibuprofen
Motrin, Motrin IB	Ibuprofen
Nalfon	Fenoprofen
Naprosyn	Naproxyn
Orudis	Ketoprofen
Rufen	Ibuprofen
Salflex	Salsalate
Tolectin	Tolmetin
Trilisate	Choline Magnesium Sodium
Voltaren	Diclofenac

*None are approved for use in pregnancy.

Table 4.4
Some Side Effects of NSAIDs

Indigestion
Heartburn
Abdominal pain
Gastritis
Peptic ulcer
Intestinal bleeding
Diarrhea
Constipation
Lowered hemoglobin (anemia)
May decrease platelet effect (important in blood clotting)
Sodium retention with edema (swelling)
Increased blood pressure (hypertension)
Abnormal liver tests (blood tests)
Can aggravate or cause kidney (renal) failure
Rash
Itching
Asthma in those allergic
Mouth ulcers
Palpitations
Dizziness
Ringing in the ears (tinnitus)
Sleepiness
Occasional blurred vision
Headaches
Confusion
Impaired thinking (uncommon, but occurs at times in older patients)
Difficulty sleeping
Depression
Fatigue
Lowered white blood count
Diminished effect of diuretics
May affect other medications taken
Sun sensitivity
Meningitis-like illness (rare)
Other individual allergic or unusual reactions

Finding a Medication Without Side Effects

Aspirin

The oldest of these drugs is aspirin. In high enough doses (usually the equivalent of 10 to 12 or more aspirins daily), aspirin can give good relief from the inflammation, pain, and swelling of arthritis. The most common side effects at this dose are upset stomach, abdominal pain, or ringing in the ears (tinnitus). The dose of aspirin is often limited by these side effects.

Aspirin can cause gastritis and peptic ulcer disease. It can also prolong bleeding by its effects on the platelets in blood. Allergic reactions, including asthma, are not common but can occur.

If aspirin is taken with a meal or antacid, then there may be less frequent indigestion, nausea, heartburn, or other stomach or abdominal side effects. Buffered aspirin or aspirin that has an antacid added may also limit these side effects. Aspirin that has a coating so that it dissolves after it has passed through the stomach may also lessen the side effects of higher doses of aspirin on the stomach.

These forms of aspirin may still produce ringing in the ears at higher doses, since this is determined by the level of aspirin in the blood. The ringing in the ears caused by aspirin goes away when the dose of aspirin is decreased or stopped.

If upset stomach, nausea, heartburn, or other abdominal discomfort happens, then you should stop the aspirin until you talk to your physician. Also, if ringing in the ears, hearing loss, or "fullness" in the head develops while taking aspirin then you should consider the possibility that it might be related to the aspirin. Talk to your physician before you continue the higher dose of aspirin product. See Table 4.5 for a list of aspirin products.

Other Noncortisone Anti-Inflammatory Drugs

Some newer medicines attempt to give the relief of pain and swelling that aspirin can give without aspirin's side effects. There are a number of these medications available, over 15 in the United States and more than 25 in other countries. Most patients

Table 4.5
Some Common Aspirin Products

Ascriptin A/D
Ascriptin (with Maalox)
Arthritis-Strength Ascriptin (with Maalox)
Arthritis-Strength Tri-Buffered Bufferin
8-Hour Bayer, Time-Release
Extra Strength Tri-Buffered Bufferin
Easprin (Enteric Coated Delayed-Release)
Empirin
Many other brand names
Zorprin (Zero-Order Release-Prolonged Action)

---

find one of these medications that gives relief with no serious side effects.

Even though up to 80 percent of people find one of this group to be effective, it is not possible to *predict* which medication will be the best for each individual. Therefore, a trial of medication is usually needed to find the "correct" one for each patient.

The correct one is the one that gives relief of pain and stiffness with no intolerable side effects. A trial of about 2 weeks is usually enough to evaluate the response. If there is not enough relief or if side effects occur then it is necessary to try a different medication.

This trial-and-error method can be frustrating to patient and physician, but is necessary to find the right medication mix for each person. A small trial size sample or prescription may help to avoid the purchase of many medications not effective or not tolerated in your case.

A list of the most commonly used of these nonsteroid anti-inflammatory drugs is in Table 4.3. Your physician can guide you as you go through the trial process.

Many people develop no side effects. If you have any side effects, they are most likely to be heartburn, indigestion, upset stomach, abdominal pain, change in bowel habits (constipation or diarrhea), gas, or other abdominal or stomach discomfort. See Table 4.4 for possible side effects.

Ulcers in the stomach or duodenum as well as irritation of the lining of the stomach can happen with any of the above feelings or without any warning signs or feelings. About 1 percent of persons using these drugs may have bleeding from the stomach or intestine the first 6 months and more may have bleeding with longer use of these medications. Older persons are at higher risk for bleeding and other problems, although everyone has some risk.

Bleeding from the stomach or intestine can be very serious so it is important to notice any new symptoms including those discussed previously. These symptoms will usually give warning to you and your physician so no serious complications happen. It is unusual but it is possible to have bleeding without any warning signs. In this case, you may notice blood in the bowel movement, the bowel movement may be black or sticky, or you may simply feel weak, dizzy, or more tired than usual. If you notice any of these signs, you should contact your physician immediately.

There are some ways to help lower the risk of irritation of the stomach and peptic ulcer disease when using anti-inflammatory drugs. The medication should be taken with food. An alternative if you are dieting is to take an antacid along with the medication to avoid the extra calories of food between meals.

Some medications can be taken to lower the risk of peptic ulcer disease and bleeding from anti-inflammatory drugs. These medications include *sucralfate (Carafate),* which is also used in the treatment of peptic ulcers. It may *directly protect the lining of the stomach* and seems especially helpful when anti-inflammatory drugs are used.

Misoprostol (Cytotec) is used to help prevent stomach (gastric) ulcers in persons who are at higher risk and must take anti-inflammatory drugs. Misoprostol has a *protection action on the stomach lining* and also decreases the production of stomach acid.

Other medications to *decrease the production of gastric acid* may also be used when taking anti-inflammatory drugs. These may help prevent stomach irritation and are also used to treat peptic ulcers. They include:

Axid (Nizatidine)
Pepcid (Famotidine)

Tagamet (Cimetidine)

Zantac (Ranitidine)

Also, antacids may be taken to *neutralize the stomach acid* which is present. This may help decrease the chance of irritation of the lining of the stomach and peptic ulcers. Some of the most common antacids are:

Amphogel	Maalox Plus
AlternaGel	Mylanta
Alu-Cap	Mylanta II
Alu-Tab	Riopan
Basaljel	Rolaids
Di-Gel	Titralac
Gelusil	Tums
Gaviscon	WinGel
Maalox	

The ideal situation is to find the anti-inflammatory drug that controls the arthritis with no side effects at all. This will minimize the need to take additional medications. However, in some cases, in order to get the benefit of the anti-inflammatory drug without side effects, it is necessary to use one or more of these additional choices. Your physician can help you decide which combination of medications is best in your own situation to help prevent irritation of the stomach and peptic ulcer disease.

If you know what to look for and do not ignore or overlook any new problem, you can be comfortable that you will discover any important side effects. If you also check with your physician at intervals for evaluation and proper blood tests, you can feel comfortable that you are monitoring adequately for side effects.

Blood tests are needed occasionally to help monitor for any unwanted effects, such as changes in the blood count, especially low hemoglobin, low white blood cells, or low platelet counts. The blood tests also check the liver and kidney function. Tests may be taken to detect small amounts of blood in the stool which can be caused by medication.

It is possible that you may have an unusual or allergic reaction to any of these medications. To be safe, if you notice any unexplained or new feeling or sign after taking a nonsteroid anti-inflammatory drug, then you should contact your physician. And, if you have had any trouble taking one of these medications, be sure to tell your physician so that precautions can be taken or medications avoided. *None should be taken during pregnancy or without your physician's knowledge.* Read the package insert about each individual medication so that you will be aware of what side effects are possible.

Medications (*analgesics*) may be needed simply to treat the pain in arthritis. This is not our first choice in pain relief, since it is better to remove the cause of the pain. But there are times, especially at first, when pain is still present before control of the arthritis is achieved. At these times, acetaminophen or aspirin in

Table 4.6
Analgesics

Trade Name	Generic Name
(See Table 4.5)	Aspirin Products
Tylenol, Anacin-3, Datril, Panadol	Acetaminophen
Motrin, Medipren, Advil, Nuprin, Rufen	Ibuprofen**
Nalfon	Fenoprofen**
Ansaid	Flurbiprofen**
Combined with other medications	Codeine**
Darvon	Propoxyphene*
Roxicodone	Oxycodone*
Talwin	Pentazocine*
Anexsia	Hydrocodone*

**Also can be used as an anti-inflammatory drug. Should *not* be used in combination with an anti-inflammatory drug without your physician's advice.
*Codeine is commonly combined with acetaminophen as Tylenol #3, Phenaphen #3, Capital and Codeine
*Propoxyphene is commonly combined with acetaminophen as Darvocet or Wygesic, or with aspirin as Darvon Compound
*Oxycodone is commonly combined with acetaminophen as Percodet, Roxicet, Tylox or combined with aspirin as Percodan.
*Pentazocine is commonly combined with acetaminophen as Talacen or with aspirin as Talwin compound.
*Hydrocodone is commonly combined with acetaminophen as Anexsia, Bancap HC, Co-Gesic, Duocet, Lorcet Plus, Lortab, Vicodin, Zydone.

Table 4.7
Some Common Muscle Relaxants

Trade Name	Generic Name
Flexeril	Cyclobenzaprine
Parafon Forte	Chlorzoxazone
Robaxin	Methocarbamol
Skelaxin	Metaxalone
Soma	Carisoprodol
Valium	Diazepam

low doses can greatly improve comfort. Occasionally stronger prescription pain medications are needed for short periods of time. These may include propoxyphene (Darvon) or codeine. The codeine is often combined with acetaminophen or aspirin. (See Table 4.6 for the most common pain medications.) Propoxyphene, codeine, oxycodone, pentazocine and hydrocodone should be used only when very necessary to avoid becoming dependent on these drugs.

Muscle Relaxants

At times, another type of medication may be used—muscle relaxants. There may be muscle spasms along with arthritis, especially when it attacks the back or neck. In some cases, in addition to the measures that treat the arthritis, a muscle relaxant may give temporary relief. In these cases, it is thought that the inflammation of arthritis causes spasm in the adjacent muscles which can be a major source of pain separate from the arthritis itself. These medications should also be minimized to avoid becoming dependent. Refer to Table 4.7 for common muscle relaxants.

Combination Treatment Is the Key

The combination of exercises, moist heat or ice, proper medication, and rest periods when needed usually improves arthritis over a period of weeks to 2 months. As activity improves and you

are able to return to your usual levels of work, it may be necessary to consider *adjusting any unusual work loads or activities.*
For example, a person with severe osteoarthritis in a knee may
need to avoid frequent stair climbing. This person would also
benefit from avoiding frequent squatting since this produces a
large amount of force on the knee. Prolonged standing or walking might also aggravate the osteoarthritis in the knee.

A person with severe arthritis in the lower back would
benefit from avoiding prolonged standing, bending, or lifting
heavy loads. All of these activities could cause a worsening of
the pain, stiffness, and limitation due to the arthritis in the spine.
In most cases, it is better to try to *adjust the work situation* to
make it more compatible with the arthritis rather than stop
working altogether.

Once there is improvement and an exercise program is
maintained, most people are able to resume a majority of their
usual daily activities. We suggest that if the regular program of
exercise is maintained along with the proper use of moist heat
and medication, that our patients gradually resume their usual
activities. As long as this regular program is continued, then
there is no limitation on activities except to avoid those which
cause severe pain. (See summary in Table 4.8.)

Table 4.8
Basic Treatment Plan

Moist heat
Exercises
Rest periods
Pace daily activities
Medications
   Anti-inflammatory drugs
      Cortisone derivatives
      Noncortisone derivatives (NSAIDs)
Analgesics if needed
Muscle relaxants if needed
Adjust unusual work loads or activities

What to Do During Flare-Ups

From time to time, there may be worsening of the pain, stiffness, and swelling. This may happen when the regular program of exercises, moist heat, and medications is not followed. It may happen after an injury, or it may just come on without any specific reason. When these "flare-ups" of arthritis begin, here are a few tips to try to regain control of the pain and stiffness.

- Be sure to give the affected joints proper rest as discussed previously.
- Use moist heat or ice packs 3 or 4 times daily for a few days.
- Begin a regular exercise program and gradually increase as discussed previously.
- Use the proper medications to help control the inflammation.

Usually these measures will regain control of the arthritis. If there is no improvement in a few days, you should contact your physician for further advice and evaluation.

There are a few warning signs that should alert you to contact your physician *earlier* than a few days since other problems may be present that require specific treatment.

Warning Signs

- An *injury* to the joint has occurred with the possibility of a fracture of a bone.
- A *fever* is present indicating that infection might need treatment.
- The pain is *very severe*.

With this program of twice daily moist heat and exercise, proper rest periods and an effective nonsteroid anti-inflammatory drug, most people are able to control the pain, stiffness, and swelling. The goal is to achieve relief of pain and to be able to continue the activities that you want to do.

Joint Protection in Arthritis

In addition to the basic treatment plan outlined so far, there are some simple actions you can take to protect your joints from needless excess forces, many of which can lead to earlier and more severe deformity. Knowing some simple techniques can greatly reduce joint stress and fatigue.

Many of the natural ways we use our hands can put stress on joints in such a way that deformity becomes more likely. For example, a tight handgrip causes forces from muscles that force the fingers in the direction of the little finger, which is a common deformity in rheumatoid arthritis.

It is important to spread the strain of work over several joints when possible. Some technical aids can greatly decrease excessive forces on joints.

Some suggestions for the *hands* include:

- *Avoid a Tight Handgrip.* Avoid carrying heavy objects by the handles (such as handbags, baskets) or using certain tools (such as scissors and pliers). A more open handgrip requires less force on the joints. Put whatever strain is necessary on the joints in such a way as to cause as little pain as possible.

- *Spread Out the Strain.* Pick up a heavy cup with two hands instead of the index finger. Instead of carrying heavy objects in your hands, when possible put them on your forearms.

- *Use "Common Sense" Aids.* A jar opener that requires little force on the fingers, and a long-handled lever for opening doors and handles puts less force on the fingers. See Table 4.10 for a list of helpful devices and aids.

- *Avoid Pressures Against the Backs of Fingers.* Pressure in this manner adds to loosening of the joints at the bases of the fingers.

- *Avoid Excessive Pressure Against the Thumb Pad.* Pinching something hard, opening a car door, and other activities such as this contribute to dislocation of the thumb.

- *Use the Strongest or Largest Joint to Do the Work.* An example of using the strongest or largest joint to do the work would be to hold a heavy bag or purse over your lower arm or shoulder rather than in your fingers.
- *Add Leverage to Reduce the Force Needed.* A leverage device that reduces the force needed for use would be a French handle on a door instead of a round door knob, or a lever on a faucet.
- *Use Lightweight Utensils When Possible.* Use lightweight utensils, cookware, and tools when possible.
- *Canes Are Useful.* With arthritis in the knee, use a cane held on the *opposite* side. Be sure the cane is the correct length. Your physician or therapist can help decide the length. Control your body weight.

In arthritis in the hip, use a cane held on the *opposite* side. Be sure the cane is the correct length. Control your body weight.

At Home and Work

- Simplify your work.
- Eliminate unnecessary steps.
- Try to decrease your demand for perfection.

Proper Foot Care Is Part of the Treatment

Proper foot care is an important part of the treatment of arthritis. As discussed in Chapter 2, many types of arthritis can cause deformities in the bones of the feet. These deformities can cause changes in the shape of the foot which result in more abnormal pressure areas, more corns and more calluses. In these cases, the foot should have a custom made shoe to avoid damage, or surgery must be considered to correct or change the deformity.

Routine Foot Care in Arthritis

Painful corns and calluses can be removed effectively, but this treatment gives only temporary relief, often 4 to 10 weeks.

This should not be done at home in "bathroom surgery." A doctor of podiatry can do this painlessly and safely. Simple removal of the corn or callus without injuring the underlying normal tissue can give immediate relief, but it may need to be repeated on a regular basis.

Home remedies for corns and calluses can greatly affect later treatment. Many preparations contain acids that do more harm than good. The use of moist heat (warm water or any of the commercial foot baths) can be helpful. If there is an open area of skin, the addition of povidone-iodine solution (such as Betadine) can be used. Water-soluble liniments such as Banalg to increase warmth, or bath oils to prevent dry skin may be helpful. Careful drying, use of skin cream, and powdering between the toes after a soak lowers the risk of dry skin and fungus infection.

Padding is available from your podiatrist or your local pharmacy. This can be temporarily effective, but avoid long-term use of any material adhered to the skin that can cause damage, especially in warm weather. Treatment with strong chemicals to remove the corn or callus is rarely effective for the long-term and can cause damage to the skin.

Orthotics

Orthotics are devices used to aid or correct an abnormality in the foot. Orthotics may be bought pre-made or may be specially adapted to a specific individual. A high quality orthotic should be custom made. Silicone materials that can be molded then activated to keep their shape may remove pressure from deformed toes. Insole types of orthotics can be made in a laboratory or custom-adapted to the foot as they are worn.

Orthotics made in a laboratory are based on an impression of the person's foot. Many materials are available, depending on the flexibility desired. A custom-made shoe insert is formed. The patient then finds a shoe that will be comfortable and able to house both the foot and the insole, which may be difficult.

A dynamic orthotic is available that allows the use of more than one pair of shoes. These are often less expensive. The insole is worn for a few days until an impression is made in the insole. Then adjustments are made as needed to give the desired effect.

Proper Shoes Are Important

Ready made shoes may not fit the foot with arthritis. "If it hurts, don't buy it." High heels and shoes with soles narrower than the width of the foot are not good for the arthritic foot. Specialized jogging and walking shoes have been an advance for the arthritic person. These shoes have more room for the foot and often have some built-in support. They are lined with softer materials and usually lace to give better support.

Some shoes are made with different shapes to actually accommodate some common deformities. For example, bunion shoes have a bulge in the place of the first toe bunion. Some shoes have extra room to accommodate an insole or other device.

Shoes should fit properly. There should be room between the end of the toes and the end of the shoe. There should be enough width to feel as though you could pinch leather across the top of the shoe at the ball of the foot. You should not be able to see the impression of your toes in the upper part of the shoe. A properly fitted shoe should not need to be "broken in."

Since the foot may change size during the day due to swelling in arthritis, shoes with laces or buckles that can be loosened may help. Shoes should be fitted at the end of the day when the swelling may be worse, then tightened in the morning.

Molded shoes are more expensive but are often the best shoes for the deformed foot. They are custom made to a complete casting of the foot. It may be less stylish than some would desire, but comfort and health may be more important!

Physical Therapy for the Feet

Physical therapy is best done for the feet on a daily basis at home when possible. Moist heat (avoiding any burning) and exercises are part of the basic treatment program of arthritis as described in Chapter 5.

Treatment of Osteoarthritis

Treatment of osteoarthritis includes a combination of exercises, rest, moist heat, or ice, as outlined in the basic treatment plan. When the treatment program is followed regularly, there is usually improvement over a few weeks to 2 months, although it will vary with the individual. Finding the most effective medication may take a trial of a few different noncortisone anti-inflammatory drugs. (See Table 4.3.) Don't be discouraged if you don't find one quickly. Each one of the entire group of medications can be effective in different persons! Your physician can guide you.

Once improvement occurs, it may not stay permanently. There may be times when osteoarthritis becomes more active again, or "flares up." This may happen when the program of exercises, moist heat, and medications is not followed regularly. It may happen after an illness or an injury, or without any specific reason. When these "flare ups" of arthritis begin, be sure that you resume regular, twice daily moist heat, twice daily exercises, and medications as you were earlier.

If the flare-up of arthritis persists despite these measures, it may be best to try a different anti-inflammatory drug. It is not known why, but at times a noncortisone anti-inflammatory drug (NSAID) may lose its effect after a period of months or years. In these cases, it is best to use a different choice from the available noncortisone anti-inflammatory drugs. Try a few others as you did earlier until you again find the "correct" one to control your joint pain and stiffness.

There are a few *warning signs* (page 59) which were outlined previously. Any of these signs should alert you to contact your physician immediately, since other problems may be present that require specific treatment. Or, if the flare-up does not improve within a few days, then it would be a good idea to contact your physician.

An option which your physician may use during a severe flare-up, depending on your own situation, is the local injection of a cortisone derivative into a joint. As discussed on page 49, these injections may offer quick improvement even though the effect may last only 6 weeks or more, depending on the severity of the arthritis and other factors.

The large majority of persons are able to control osteoarthritis with this simple program. The goal is to allow you to have relief of pain and stiffness and to allow the activities which you feel are necessary. If you do not find enough improvement or if pain continues to be constant and intolerable, talk with your physician about the possibility of treatment of the osteoarthritis with surgery.

Treatment of Bursitis

Treatment of bursitis usually includes moist heat such as a hot shower, hot bathtub, whirlpool, or hot towels. These steps are outlined in the basic treatment program in Table 4.8. Other methods such as a moist heating pad or additional procedures are also available. Moist heat for 10 to 20 minutes twice daily or trying an ice pack for a similar time is recommended. As the pain decreases, exercises are added to increase the flexibility and improve the strength of the surrounding muscles. Exercises prevent longer lasting or even permanent loss of movement in the affected area such as the shoulder. It is helpful to see a physical therapist at first if movement is very painful and limited.

Your physician may suggest an anti-inflammatory medication to help decrease the pain and allow more effective exercises. If the pain is severe or persistent, a local injection into the bursa with a cortisone derivative may be given. This injection usually gives quick and effective relief. It is important to remember that bursitis does improve and is not usually a severely limiting or crippling problem over a long period.

Treatment of Tendinitis

Treatment of tendinitis may include the use of rest, moist heat, or ice as in bursitis above and a careful exercise program to improve the flexibility and strength of the surrounding muscles. The basic treatment plan outlines these steps in Table 4.8.

At times, anti-inflammatory medications may help although in severe tendinitis at the elbow and other areas, medicines taken by mouth often do not seem to be very effective. Local injections into the area with a cortisone derivative and occasionally surgery may be necessary. This depends a lot on the individual situation so that your physician can guide you.

Avoidance of frequent repetitive use of the muscle and a regular exercise program may help prevent a recurrence of the tendinitis.

Treatment of Fibrositis (Fibromyalgia)

Fibrositis may be a chronic illness and the various treatments may not always be successful. We suggest a regular program of moist heat twice daily as part of the basic treatment program. The exercises should involve the neck, back, shoulders, hips, knees, and other areas of discomfort. Those patients who can maintain a regular program of exercise have more relief of pain on a regular basis. A trial of a few different anti-inflammatory drugs is helpful. Many people find quite a bit of relief from these medications.

If you do not feel there has been enough improvement with the steps taken in the basic treatment program, there are other medications and treatment available. These are discussed on page 144.

In this group of arthritis-related problems, the patients who control their pain and regain control of their lives are those who are able to keep up the regular program of twice daily moist heat, twice daily exercises, and finding the proper combination of medication.

Most people who follow this program find improvement. As the pain and stiffness improve, many people are able to decrease their medication or stop it altogether. If you know what to do, you can control this just as you can manage other parts of your life.

Rheumatoid Arthritis

Treatment of rheumatoid arthritis begins with moist heat twice daily, just as in other types of arthritis. This is even more important in rheumatoid arthritis because there is active inflammation of the joints. The steps for the basic treatment plan are outlined in Table 4.8. The heat helps decrease the swelling and stiffness to allow exercise and use of the joints. Moist heat is usually most effective. This can be achieved using a shower, bathtub, whirlpool, hot towels, moist heating pad, or other methods.

It takes up to 2 months for the average person to feel a response from the heat and exercise. This means that you may do all the right things for days or weeks with little or no noticeable improvement. This may lead to discouragement and may cause you to stop the regular program. It might be necessary for you to talk to your physician or physical therapist during this time to keep yourself on the right course.

One thing is definite—those who improve are those who are able to maintain a regular exercise program. And those who don't maintain a regular program usually don't get that initial improvement.

Anti-inflammatory medications are very useful in rheumatoid arthritis. The majority of people do find one of the nonsteroid anti-inflammatory drugs (NSAIDS) available that gives adequate control of joint pain and swelling. When there is improvement in joint pain and swelling, there is usually also improvement in fatigue and in morning stiffness.

There is no magic or scientific way to predict which medication will be the "correct" one for each person. It is necessary to try them one at a time and judge how effective they are. If there is no improvement, then try a different medication. You should expect to find good relief of pain and stiffness.

Try each medication for about 2 weeks and make a decision on its effectiveness. Occasionally a response may take longer but if there is no effect at all during this time then the medication is not likely to be the "correct" one.

Despite the frequent warnings we hear, the fact is that most persons do not have severe side effects from this group of drugs. However, caution is still needed as long as you require these medications. Every medication has benefits and risks. The possible side effects of these drugs are reviewed in Table 4.4. If the benefits outweigh the risks, then the drug may be taken. If the risks are greater than any potential benefit, then the drug should be avoided.

Most persons find at least one of these medications which gives relief in rheumatoid arthritis without side effects. If you try the 15 or more available, it is likely that one or more will give enough improvement to continue.

If you notice no side effects, your physician can help you monitor for other detectable problems on occasional visits at intervals of a few months. Blood tests are needed at times to be sure there are no side effects on the blood, kidney, liver, or other internal organs. If any problems are detected, they are usually quickly reversible by decreasing the dosage or stopping the medication. It is very unusual to require any additional medications or treatment for the side effects detected through blood tests.

The strongest anti-inflammatory drugs are in the cortisone group. These drugs are strong enough that for many persons they can give almost complete relief of the pain and swelling of rheumatoid arthritis. The problem is that in high doses over a long period, these drugs can have severe long-term side effects. Also, these drugs do not slow down the progress of rheumatoid arthritis. The destructive or crippling effects of the arthritis will not be stopped. As soon as the drug is stopped, the arthritis may return as severe as it was earlier plus any side effects that have developed.

However, the cortisone drugs can be used effectively in rheumatoid arthritis. They can be used in *low doses* to gain control in severe cases, especially when the alternative is severe incapacitation or loss of job or family. This is especially helpful when one of the slower-acting drugs is started. The patient gets quick improvement from the low dose of cortisone and has a good chance for long-term control of the disease from the second drug. When improvement begins, the cortisone drug is gradually stopped. These low doses usually have minimal side effects when used for a short period of time.

Another use of cortisone derivatives in rheumatoid arthritis is in local injections into joints. This gives good, quick relief that usually lasts for 4 to 8 weeks or more depending on the severity of the rheumatoid arthritis. Local injection is used when one or two joints are much more severely affected than others. It can also be used when other treatment has worked except in one or

Table 4.9
Some Common Suppressive or Disease-Modifying Drugs

Gold Compounds	
Capsules	
Auranofin	Ridaura
Injections	
Gold Sodium Thiomalate	Myochrysine
Aurothioglucose	Solganal
Methotrexate	
Tablets	Rheumatrex
Injections	Methotrexate
Penicillamine	
Tablets	Depen
Capsules	Cuprimine
Sulfasalazine (not formally approved by Food and Drug Administration for use in Rheumatoid Arthritis)	
Tablets	Azulfidine
Azathioprine	
Tablets	Imuran
Hydroxychloroquine	
Tablets	Plaquenil
Cyclophosphamide (not formally approved by Food and Drug Administration for use in Rheumatoid Arthritis)	
Tablets	Cytoxan
Chlorambucil (not used frequently—not formally approved by Food and Drug Administration for use in Rheumatoid Arthritis)	
Tablets	Leukeran

two joints. Serious side effects of the local injection into the joint are rare but infection can occur. Occasionally pain and swelling may become worse for 1 or 2 days immediately after an injection, then relief follows. In 5 to 10 percent of cases, the injection does not give very much relief.

It is not always easy to decide whether there has been enough improvement with the basic program of moist heat, exercises, rest and anti-inflammatory medications since there may be partial relief. We feel that there should be enough improvement that a person is comfortable and able to do the activities they feel necessary. This will be different for each person. Don't be hesitant to let your physician know if you do not feel adequate improvement.

The improvement in rheumatoid arthritis usually happens over a few months with the basic treatment program. As long as there is steady progress, it is usually a good idea to continue the same treatment to see what total improvement occurs. If the final level of improvement is not acceptable, then there is another group of medicines that offers a good chance of excellent results.

In rheumatoid arthritis, about 20 percent or more of patients may not have enough benefit and improvement from the program outlined so far. Or, you may not tolerate an anti-inflammatory drug that could be effective for you. In these cases, a second group of medications is available that attempts to suppress the arthritis and better control the disease activity. These are called suppressive or disease-modifying drugs.

Each of this group of medications may give improvement in 50 percent or more of persons who take them. Some have up to an 80 percent chance of improvement. Up to 30 percent of those who improve may have their arthritis go into remission, which means most signs of the arthritis disappear or become very well controlled. It is possible that some of these medications may slow the entire progress of the arthritis, especially when this remission is achieved.

If these are such effective medications, why don't we use them on all rheumatoid arthritis patients? Most patients do well enough without these medications. They take much longer to work—the average time of response to these medications is 6 to 12 weeks or longer. Also, they have some potential side effects that require regular testing. And finally, patients and physicians generally prefer to use the least number of medications possible.

These suppressive or disease-modifying drugs have some similarities even though they are each very different medications. The exact way in which they work to improve rheumatoid arthritis is not known. They are all slow acting, usually requiring

at least 6 weeks to notice any improvement (but commonly requiring 10 or more weeks). From 50 to 80 percent of people with
this disease have improvement and up to 30 percent of those
who improve have excellent relief of most symptoms of rheumatoid arthritis. For many people, the patience to continue a regular
program of treatment is well rewarded with an excellent result
and control of arthritis when one of these drugs is added.

The choice of medications depends on each individual situation. You and your physician must take into account other medications taken, any earlier problems taking medications, and other
factors. Table 4.9 lists some of the most commonly used medications in this group of drugs. Since there are a number of choices
in this group, the large majority of patients are able to gain good
control of their rheumatoid arthritis.

Splints Used for Quick Improvement

Splints can be an important part of the treatment program
in rheumatoid arthritis. When arthritis is acute with severe pain
on movement of a joint, a splint can give quick improvement
in pain. Splints are also used in more severe long-lasting cases of
arthritis to try to prevent deformity.

The most common splints used in rheumatoid arthritis are
for the hands and wrists. These splints have several purposes.

Hand and wrist splints can protect weak muscles, ligaments, and swollen, painful joints caused by the arthritis.

These splints support the hands and wrists by immobilizing
the joints and forcing them to rest. This allows much faster relief
when arthritis is severe. It allows these joints to have rest while a
person is otherwise active.

Hand and wrist splints attempt to prevent deformity by sta-
bilizing a joint and holding it in proper position. This also helps
the patient learn to hold the joints in the proper position when
the splint is not being worn.

Today's splints are neat, trim, lightweight, and durable.
They are usually secured with velcro straps and are easily put on
and off. Today's splints are kept clean easily and are relatively

inexpensive. Splints are like new shoes. They are designed and fitted to each person as an individual.

The occupational therapist is the person who is trained in the proper construction and demonstration of the use of splints. You and your physician can decide on the best splint to achieve the desired purpose.

Three of the most commonly used splints for the hands and wrists in rheumatoid arthritis are the *resting splint,* the *dynamic or working splint,* and the *ulnar drift splint.*

The resting or static splint can support the entire hand and wrist in a position which is properly aligned and comfortable (see Figure 4.3). The thumb, wrist, and fingers are all supported in a proper position. These splints are usually worn at night and help alleviate pain. They may be worn during the day, but they prevent movement of the joints. When arthritis is acute or severe, these splints can help bring pain relief faster by resting the joints.

Dynamic or working splints give firm wrist support in a comfortable position. This splint allows the fingers and thumb to move freely (see Figure 4.4). It can be worn on the job when only wrist support is needed.

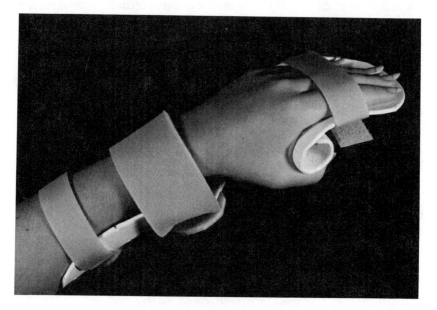

Figure 4.3. A resting splint.

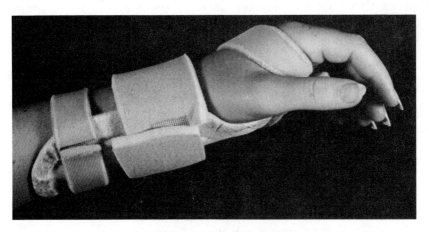

Figure 4.4. A working splint.

Ulnar drift splints are for those patients whose fingers are beginning to drift or deviate toward the little finger (see Figure 4.5). This is a common situation in rheumatoid arthritis that has been present over a long period of time. There are several new, soft ulnar drift splints available now that support and align the fingers in a proper position.

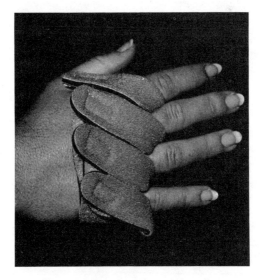

Figure 4.5. An ulnar drift splint.

Other common devices used by people with rheumatoid arthritis to make daily activities easier include some very practical ideas. There are many aids available depending on the needs of each patient.

For example, a toilet seat extension can be used to make sitting and arising from the toilet easier and less painful. Several can and jar openers are simple to install and use. These devices take work loads off those inflamed joints for better long-term joint protection. Table 4.10 is a list of some of the most common and most useful devices and aids.

Table 4.10
Some Common and Useful Devices Available

Grips for pens and pencils
Pens shaped for arthritic hands
Reachers of all sizes to grip objects, pick up off the floor
Soft tubes to enlarge the grip of brush and comb
Buttoning and zipping device for use with only one closed hand
Bottle and jar opener for use with one hand
Device to turn handles and knobs
Devices and dishes to prevent spilling and make pouring easy
Utensils and holders which can be used with a hand without
    the assistance of the fingers
Shower and bath chairs, stools, and rails
Raised toilet seats
Canes, walkers with or without rollers
Lifter seat
Chair back support
Chair leg extenders
Embroidery loop and needle holder
Non-slip bath mattress
Shoelace fasteners
Device for putting on socks without bending
Exercise mat
Two-handed knife
Car door opener for one hand
Non-slip cane attachment
Device to help put on trousers
Exercise Aids

Shoes Must Fit Correctly

Proper shoes are important to the feet of rheumatoid arthritis patients. Shoes must fit correctly and give enough support. Shoes that are correct can make a major difference in comfort and ability to walk.

The most common problem in rheumatoid arthritis is the need for wider or deeper shoes to give enough room for the toes and front part of the foot. Most ready-made shoes are not built in this way. If you are unable to locate proper shoes, it may be necessary to have shoes made specially. Other adjustments for the shoe can be made to make walking more comfortable and to prevent future damage to the foot. Your physician or podiatrist can advise you.

Outline the Best Program to Win with Rheumatoid Arthritis

To beat rheumatoid arthritis, each person must make a plan. Talk with your physician and outline the best program to allow you to gain control over the pain and regain the activities you desire. Then follow the program. Those who maintain a program of heat and exercises combined with the most effective medications can control the active arthritis. For long-term control to limit deformities and loss of use of the joints, some people may need other plans including splints and surgical treatment. It can be frustrating, but the relief of pain and the improvement in activity and use of the joints is worth the time and effort. If you have the facts, you can take an active part in your own treatment plan.

Surgery may be a necessary alternative for treatment of rheumatoid arthritis. This is discussed on page 145.

Systemic Lupus Erythematosus (SLE or Lupus)

In systemic lupus erythematosus (SLE or lupus), many patients do well if they maintain the basic treatment plan outlined in Table 4.8. A program of heat and exercises, non-steroid anti-inflammatory drugs, and use of the lowest possible dose of one of the cortisone derivatives when necessary usually allows good control of the disease.

Treatment of lupus includes moist heat and exercises for the joints to keep them flexible and to strengthen muscles. This is followed just as described for rheumatoid arthritis. The combination of twice daily moist heat and exercises when arthritis is active is very important in lupus. The time and effort involved will be worth the improvement, but it may take weeks or months to see the effect.

Proper rest is important in lupus, especially when fatigue is prominent. A 20 to 30 minute rest period late in the morning and late in the afternoon may be even more important in lupus than in rheumatoid arthritis. This greatly helps the energy during the rest of the day. It is usually appreciated by both patient and family. Ten hours of bedrest (it is not necessary to sleep the entire time) is also important when the disease is more active.

Anti-inflammatory medications help control the joint pain and stiffness and may help improve the fatigue. Nonsteroid anti-inflammatory drugs (NSAIDS) are usually tried first. These medications do not cure lupus but there is usually one that does help control symptoms. It is important to watch for side effects when these are used in lupus, just as in other types of arthritis.

When noncortisone anti-inflammatory drugs are not enough, the cortisone derivatives such as prednisone may be helpful in lupus. These are used mainly when there is internal organ disease such as kidney disease, heart disease, brain disease, lung disease, and blood disorders. Much higher doses may be required than in rheumatoid arthritis, up to 20 to 60 mg of prednisone daily. The side effects of higher doses of the cortisone derivatives may present more problems including weight gain, fullness in the face, bone thinning (osteoporosis), fractures of bones, and diabetes mellitus (high blood glucose). When these medications are used, there is always an attempt to use the lowest possible dose for the shortest possible time to keep side effects at the lowest level.

If anti-inflammatory medications are not enough to control the disease, there are other medications that help to suppress lupus, especially when there is internal organ disease. These drugs that suppress the disease are also often used when high doses of cortisone drugs are needed over a long time. By adding one of these "suppressive" drugs, it is often possible to lower or stop altogether the cortisone derivatives. There are other ways that you and your physician may be able to control or limit many of the side effects of the needed cortisone treatment.

These suppressive drugs may also have side effects. Although each person is different and each medication is different, some common side effects include rash, nausea and other stomach and intestine-related discomfort, blood disorders, and kidney and bladder problems. These side effects are usually able to be managed as long as each person takes the responsibility of monitoring the drug.

Monitoring the drug includes knowing the side effects, reporting any new problems to your physician, and keeping up with regular blood tests and other laboratory monitoring. Table 4.9 lists some of the most commonly used drugs of this type. A detailed list of possible side effects is available in the Physicians' Desk Reference (PDR) published yearly, but for a practical guide to the side effects *you* should be most concerned about, talk with your physician. Remember, every medication has benefits and risks, and the benefits should outweigh the risks for you.

Systemic lupus erythematosus in years past had a high mortality. Better methods with earlier diagnosis and more effective treatment have changed that situation. Most patients may now expect to live a normal lifetime with careful treatment and follow-up by their physician. Most persons who suffer from lupus have times of discouragement and depression. It is important to have someone to talk with such as a family member, minister, friend, psychologist, or psychiatrist. In many areas, there are groups which meet to share concerns and share emotional support. These groups can be a great source of comfort by sharing experiences, as discussed in Chapter 10.

If you know the facts, you can be more effective in controlling the problems which lupus can bring. You can also be an active part of the treatment plan along with your physician.

Juvenile Rheumatoid Arthritis

The basic treatment program (Table 4.8) is usually effective in juvenile rheumatoid arthritis. There is generally a response to treatment and many children have improvement so that signs and feelings of the arthritis become minimized or a remission occurs.

However, in some cases, the arthritis may continue to be limiting or may be severe enough to need a cortisone derivative such as prednisone for control. In these cases, a second medication from the "suppressive" group of drugs used in adult rheumatoid arthritis may be helpful. This may allow better control of the arthritis. It may allow the cortisone derivative to be stopped, or at least used in the lowest possible dose.

Since these patients are younger, the use of any medication must be even more careful than in adults. Some of the suppressive drugs have been used more widely in children than others. When parents and physician monitor the medication and its effects then one of these can usually be given without side effects to allow better control of the disease. This may also make it possible to delay the progress of the disease itself.

Ankylosing Spondylitis

Treatment of ankylosing spondylitis includes moist heat twice daily just as discussed for rheumatoid arthritis. An exercise program is extremely important in ankylosing spondylitis. Exercises are best done while using heat such as a shower, bathtub, hot towels, or pool. Proper back exercises are the very best way to prevent the back from becoming stooped over. It may not be possible to prevent stiffness, but if the posture is maintained even a stiff spine will not be as limiting. Many professionals and others work and live a quite normal life with severe stiffness in the spine if the posture is maintained.

Specific exercises are helpful to maintain correct posture as well as to strengthen the muscles of the back. Swimming is an excellent exercise since it strengthens the muscles of the back with little stress on the joints. Running or jogging should be avoided since this puts more stress on the joints of the back. The exercises in Chapter 5 are an excellent basis for a program for ankylosing spondylitis.

Anti-inflammatory medications often control the pain and stiffness of ankylosing spondylitis. One of the nonsteroid anti-inflammatory drugs (NSAIDS) usually gives control of pain and allows exercise and activity. Indomethacin, sulindac, naproxen, diclofenac, or aspirin are often helpful. However, as in other types of arthritis remember that a large majority of persons find ONE of this entire group of medications which gives good relief of pain and stiffness with no unwanted side effects. If one does not give adequate relief then try a different one, as described for rheumatoid arthritis. Be alert for possible side effects to prevent problems arising from medication.

Ankylosing spondylitis is important to detect and treat since most arthritis specialists feel so much can be done to prevent limitation and deformity. This arthritis can be managed if the facts are known and an effective plan is made for control of the pain and stiffness and for proper, regular exercises. If this is continued then you should expect to continue to live a near-normal life without worries about future crippling and deformity. It is especially important to maintain strength and flexibility in the back, the neck, the hips, and the shoulders in ankylosing spondylitis, since these are the most commonly affected joints. Certain specific exercises from Chapter 5 should be included in a regular basic treatment program. These include:

- Neck exercises
- Shoulder exercises
- Hip exercises
- Back exercises
- Deep breathing exercises
- Posture exercises

Posture is important in ankylosing spondylitis. Proper posture will help prevent permanent stiffness in a position that is limiting. For example, in years past, people with ankylosing spondylitis developed a posture which was bent over and stiffened, making it very difficult to carry out daily activities. With proper posture, exercises, and treatment, many men and women are able to continue near normal occupations, social and athletic activities.

There are a few important suggestions for maintaining posture in ankylosing spondylitis.

- Don't slump. Sit with your back firmly against the back of the chair. A lumbar support or a rolled up towel in the lower part of the back may help keep the spine in its natural position.
- Sit in a chair that allows your feet to rest on the floor with hips level.
- Try not to lean forward at the hips when sitting at a desk or while driving.
- Try to alternate sitting with standing and walking to prevent stiffness in the hips and back.
- Try to sleep on a firm mattress. It is a good idea to spend at least part of the night without a pillow under your head. A rolled up towel may be useful to support the normal curve in the neck. Try not to use pillows under your legs when sleeping on your back. Also, try to spend at least part of the night sleeping on your stomach.

Gout

The acute attack of gout is treated with one of the nonsteroid anti-inflammatory drugs a medicine called colchicine. Most commonly used are indomethacin, naproxen, or others. Colchicine has been used for many years and remains a good treatment, although diarrhea is common when pills are taken in higher doses. Relief usually comes within a day or two although the entire attack may last longer. Occasionally a cortisone derivative may be used.

After diagnosis, medications are available which can help prevent future attacks of gout and uric acid kidney stones. These include allopurinol (Zyloprim), which decreases the production of uric acid by the body. Probenecid (Benemid) increases the removal of uric acid from the blood by the kidneys. Both of these medications lower the blood level of uric acid to reduce and usually totally eliminate attacks.

For the first few months, indomethacin, naproxen, colchicine, or other medication is added to prevent acute attacks.

Much is said about diet in gout. If your diet is high in meats, protein, and organ meats such as liver, kidney, and brain, then it is helpful to decrease these foods. If you drink alcohol in large amounts then it will help to limit your intake. The average American diet is otherwise not a major problem in producing gout. The need for a very strict diet is not as strong today because the medications are so effective.

Gout is one kind of arthritis which is able to be controlled completely in most cases by medication. This makes it an important problem to recognize since it is so treatable. This is one kind of arthritis you do NOT have to "live with."

Psoriatic Arthritis

The basic treatment program for psoriatic arthritis is often successful in controlling the pain, stiffness and swelling. When heat, exercises and nonsteroid anti-inflammatory drugs are not enough for good control then some of the same drugs used to control severe rheumatoid arthritis are helpful. One of this group of suppressive drugs, Table 4.9, can offer improvement in the arthritis and may help delay the progress and crippling of the arthritis.

Methotrexate and gold are the most commonly used of this group of medications in psoriatic arthritis. Their use is usually similar as in rheumatoid arthritis. The rash of psoriasis should also be treated and controlled as well as possible.

Polymyalgia Rheumatica

Treatment usually requires low doses of prednisone or other cortisone derivative. There is usually very quick improvement and return to feeling nearly normal over days. Then the medication is slowly decreased over a period of months as long as improvement continues. There are usually no permanent effects of the polymyalgia rheumatica such as crippling or deformity after it leaves.

Temporal Arteritis

Treatment requires prednisone or other cortisone derivative. The dose is higher than in polymyalgia rheumatica, but there is usually a very quick improvement. Then the dose of prednisone is gradually decreased over a period of many months as long as improvement continues. If treated early, there are usually no permanent complications of temporal arteritis but the prednisone required may cause some side effects of its own. Many of these may be able to be controlled or prevented with your physician's help.

Scleroderma

The cause of scleroderma is not known, and there is no sure treatment. Moist heat and exercises are used to preserve the use of the hands and other joints. Skin care must be immaculate to prevent infections. When the disease affects the kidneys, heart, lungs, esophagus, or other internal organs treatment directed at the specific problem is used. There are a number of medications used to attempt to change the skin thickening and tightening, but none so far has been shown to have excellent results.

Sjogren's Syndrome

There is no really good treatment for Sjogren's syndrome. Fortunately, most people with rheumatoid arthritis who are affected by Sjogren's syndrome have mild symptoms mainly limited to dryness in the eyes or dryness in the mouth. The dryness in the eyes is treated with artificial tears which lubricate the eyes to prevent infection and scarring. In severe cases, other treatment may be needed by your opthamologist.

The mouth dryness is treated by using frequent sips of water or other liquids and careful dental care. Liquids are available over the counter to help lubricate the mouth. Since there is less normal saliva to help prevent cavities, special attention to dental condition is needed including proper cleaning and the use of fluoride toothpaste, mouthwash, or applications as suggested by your dentist. A form of electrical stimulation has been used recently with success in some cases of mouth dryness.

CHAPTER FIVE

Exercises for Strength and Mobility

Exercises are one of the best long-term ways to increase the strength in your muscles and give you more mobility with your arthritis. In our clinic, we find that people with all types of arthritis who begin and maintain an adequate exercise program are almost always able to see and feel improvement. On the other hand, those persons who do not use exercise as part of their treatment for arthritis usually find much less relief from the pain and stiffness.

In starting an exercise program as part of your basic treatment plan, you must allow yourself time to get adjusted to the movements, to learn the exercises, and to condition your body to perform each exercise in a manner that will increase your strength. It usually requires weeks to learn the exercises effectively and to be able to perform the correct number of repetitions twice daily. But with a strong commitment and will to succeed, almost every person with arthritis can successfully follow the program. Your physical therapist is a specialist trained to help you accomplish this goal.

Remember to begin slowly with only 1 or 2 repetitions of each exercise twice daily—usually in the morning and each evening. Gradually increase until you can work up to 10, then up to 20 repetitions of each exercise twice daily. If you have more pain after you exercise, you may need to begin again doing only 1 or 2 of the first exercise once a day and *gradually* increase.

Do not be concerned if you can only do one repetition of the first exercise as you start your program. You should have no more pain after you finish than when you started your exercises. If you experience severe pain while exercising, you should stop. Then at the next session, try one or two of the exercises. When you have mastered this number, try three or four repetitions, gradually increasing the number of exercises and repetitions. The goal—10 to 20 of each exercise twice daily—is the level that seems to work well to maintain the highest level of strength and flexibility.

Some days you will not feel like exercising, especially when you are uncomfortable or tired. But you must begin a regular and compulsive program of twice daily exercise to be done every day—good days and bad days as well—in order to achieve maximum improvement with your arthritis. When your arthritis improves, don't stop the regular exercise program.

Let's review the specific exercises that can allow you to maintain joint flexibility and muscle strength (Figures 5.1–5.5).

Neck Mobility and Flexibility

These exercises improve the mobility and flexibility of the neck. Flexibility helps your body perform more effectively. You may do these sitting or standing, whichever is more comfortable for you. Some people like to do these exercises in front of a mirror. Keep your head straight and looking forward. Try to achieve the most movement possible with the range of motion exercises. Then try the isometric strengthening exercises. These should begin with minimal resistance, very gradually increasing the resistance as you are able. Sometimes it is helpful to have some gentle assistance from a family member or friend. Your physical therapist can show you how.

Range of Motion

Flexion

Look down and bend the chin forward to the chest (see figure 5.1). If you feel stiffness or pain, do not force the movement. Go as far as you can move easily. If pain persists with this or any exercise then stop until you have talked to your physician or physical therapist.

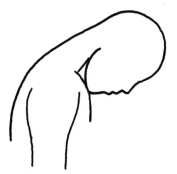

Figure 5.1.   A flexion exercise.

Extension

Look up and bend the head back as far as possible without forcing any movement (see Figure 5.2). If you feel pain or dizziness, stop until you talk to your physician or physical therapist.

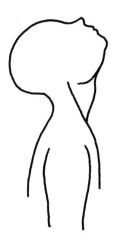

Figure 5.2.   An extension exercise.

Lateral Flexion

Tilt the left ear to the left shoulder (but do not raise the shoulder). If you feel pain or resistance, do not force the motion.

Now tilt the right ear to the right shoulder just as you did for the left ear. (See Figure 5.3.)

Figure 5.3.   A lateral flexion exercise.

Rotation

Turn to look over your left shoulder. Try to make your chin even with your shoulder. Go as far as is comfortable, but do not force the movement. (See Figure 5.4.)

Now turn and look over your right shoulder, just as you did for the left shoulder.

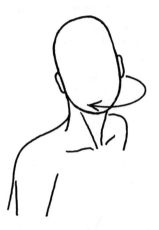

Figure 5.4.   A rotation exercise.

Neck Isometric Exercises

Neck isometric exercises are more advanced exercises to help strengthen the muscles of the neck. Try these gently and gradually after range of motion of the neck is improved as much as possible.

Isometric Flexion

Place hand on your forehead. Try to look down while resisting the motion with your hand. Hold for 6 seconds. Count out loud. *Do not* hold your breath. (See Figure 5.5.)

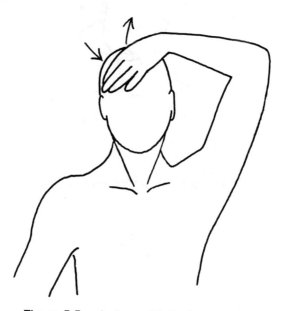

Figure 5.5.   An isometric flexion exercise.

Isometric Extension

Place your hands on the back of your head. (See Figure 5.6.) Try to look up and back while resisting the motion with your hands. Hold for 6 seconds. Count out loud. *Do not* hold your breath.

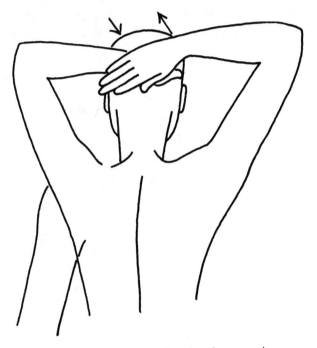

Figure 5.6.   An isometric extension exercise.

Isometric Lateral Flexion

Start with your head straight. Place your left hand just above your left ear. (See Figure 5.7.) Try to tilt your head to the left but resist the motion with your left hand. Hold for 6 seconds. Count out loud. *Do not* hold your breath.

Now place your right hand just above your right ear. Try to tilt your head to the right but resist the movement with your right hand. Hold for 6 seconds. Count out loud. *Do not* hold your breath.

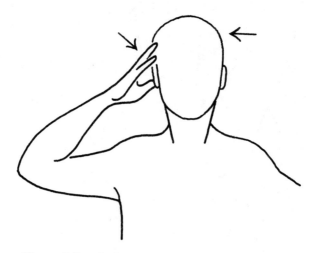

Figure 5.7.　An isometric lateral flexion exercise.

Isometric Rotation

Place your left hand above your ear and near your left fore-head. (See Figure 5.8.) Now try to look over your left shoulder but resist the motion with your left hand. (The hand should not be placed lower on the jaw.) Hold for 6 seconds. Count out loud. *Do not* hold your breath.

Place your right hand above your ear and near your right forehead. Now try to look over your right shoulder but resist the motion with your right hand. Hold for 6 seconds. Count out loud. *Do not* hold your breath.

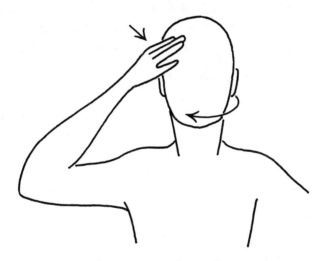

Figure 5.8.   An isometric rotation exercise.

Shoulder Exercises

Shoulder Flexibility

These exercises will increase the flexibility of the shoulders and arms. Increasing the number of exercises can increase the strength of the arms.

Shoulder External Rotation

These exercises increase the motion you use to comb your hair. You may sit, stand, or lie down to do these exercises. (See Figure 5.9.)

Clasp your hands behind your head. Pull your elbows together until they are as close as possible in front of your chin. Separate the elbows out to the side as much as possible.

Repeat this, gradually increasing to 5, then 10, then up to 20 repetitions. You may repeat these 2 or 3 times daily.

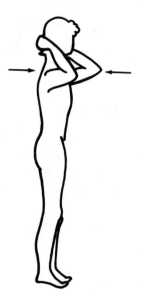

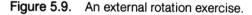

Figure 5.9. An external rotation exercise.

Shoulder Internal Rotation

These exercises increase the flexibility of the shoulders in the motions women use to fasten a bra in the back or men use to put a wallet in a back pocket. This exercise is best done standing and is often done in the shower using a wash cloth to wash your upper back and a towel to dry it. (See Figure 5.10.)

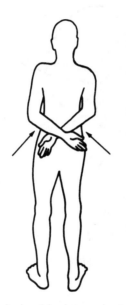

Figure 5.10.   A shoulder internal rotation exercise.

Shoulder Flexion

Shoulder flexion is the exercise you do when you raise your arms straight overhead. (See Figure 5.11.)

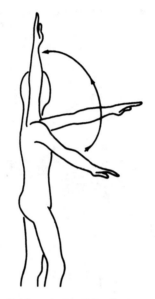

Figure 5.11.   A shoulder flexion exercise.

Shoulder Abduction

Shoulder abduction is raising the arms straight out away from your side and up above your head. Try this with your palm up. If your arms hurt or if you have difficulty raising them straight over your head when sitting or standing, try lying on your bed and holding a stick (a broom handle will do).

1. Now raise your arms, keeping them straight and holding the stick with both hands, up over your head as far as possible. The less painful arm will help the painful arm go further.
2. Repeat this exercise, gradually increasing to 5, then 10, then 20 repetitions two or three times a day.
3. Now raise your arms out to the side, one at a time, and slowly make big circles. (See Figure 5.12.)
4. Repeat this exercise, gradually increasing to 5, then 10, then 20 repetitions two or three times a day.

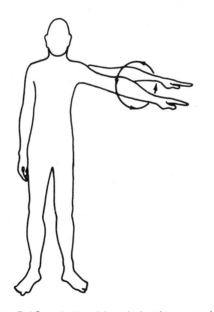

Figure 5.12.   A shoulder abduction exercise.

Shoulder Girdle Rotation

This exercise can be done in a sitting or standing position and is fun to do during the day to relieve neck and shoulder tension and maintain shoulder girdle flexibility. (See Figure 5.13.)

1. Roll your shoulders in a forward circle, raise shoulders towards the ears in a shrugging motion. Roll shoulders back and chest out as in a military stance. Lower the shoulders and bring the shoulders forward. Think of it as a simple shoulder roll in a circle. Now reverse the process, rolling your shoulder girdle in a backward circle.
2. Repeat this exercise, gradually increasing to 5, then 10, then 20 repetitions two or three times a day if possible.

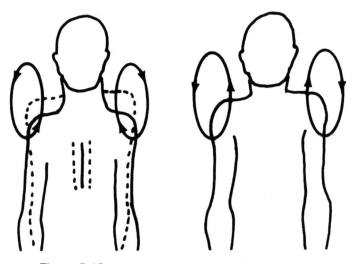

Figure 5.13.   A shoulder girdle rotation exercise.

Elbow and Arm Exercises

Elbow Flexion and Extension

Bend each elbow, bringing the hand toward the top of the shoulder and then straighten the arm completely, moving it to the side of your body. Be sure to extend the arm fully to the body to gain full motion. Repeat this 5, then 10, then 20 times two or three times each day.

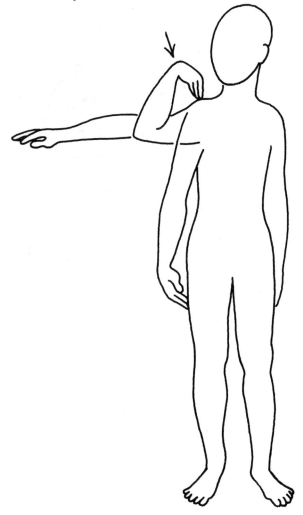

Figure 5.14. An elbow flexion and extension exercise.

Forearm Pronation and Supination

Turn each palm up then turn the palm down. Keep the elbows beside your waist. Repeat this 5, then 10, then 20 times two or three times each day.

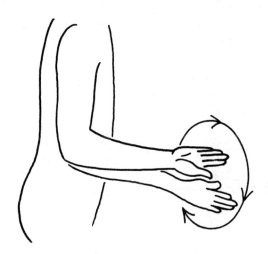

Figure 5.15.   A pronation and supination exercise.

Wrist, Hand, and Finger Exercises

Wrist Flexion and Extension

To maintain mobility and flexibility in the wrists, use the other hand to bend the wrist gently as far as possible. Support your arm on a table or on the arm of a chair. Avoid holding the arm in mid-air when doing these exercises. (See Figure 5.16.)

Place one hand over the edge of a table and use the other hand to first bend the hand up as far as possible, then bend the hand down as far as possible.

Bend the hand as far as you can bend easily. Repeat this, gradually increasing up to 5, then 10, then 20 repetitions each session. Repeat the session two times each day.

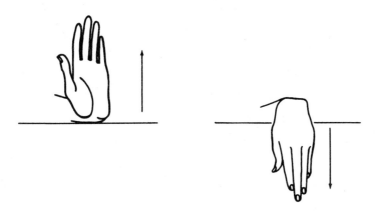

Figure 5.16.   A wrist flexion and extension exercise.

Wrist Ulnar and Radial

Place your hand palm down on a table. Slide fingers and hand toward thumb using other hand to assist as needed. Do not move elbow.

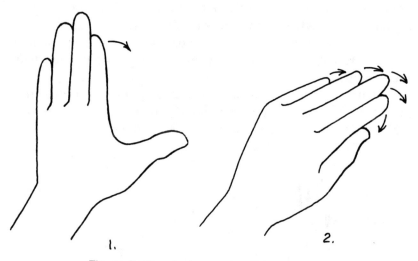

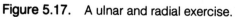

Figure 5.17.   A ulnar and radial exercise.

Finger Flexion and Extension

Close your fingers and make a fist. Then open the fist, extending the fingers as straight as possible. Repeat 5 times, gradually increasing to 10 and then 20 times twice daily.

Use a foam or sponge ball (such as a Nerf ball), slightly larger than the size of a tennis ball, and squeeze and release for this exercise. Make sure all your fingers close as far as possible around the ball. Release and straighten the fingers. It is important to use a foam rather than a hard rubber ball. Foam balls are available at toy stores. (See Figure 5.18.)

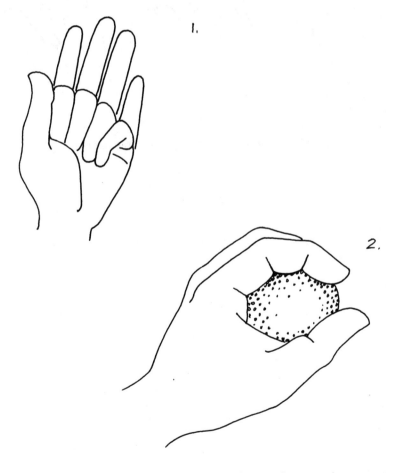

Figure 5.18.   A finger flexion and extension exercise.

Assisted Finger Flexion

Curling each finger down, bend each joint in the finger as far as possible. The other hand may be used to assist the fingers gently. Do not force movement if it is painful. Repeat for each finger 5, then 10, then 20 times twice daily. (See Figure 5.19.)

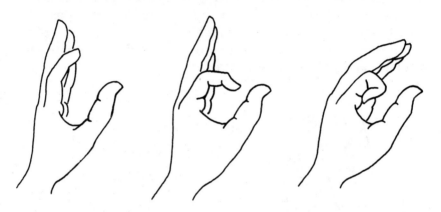

Figure 5.19.   An assisted finger flexion exercise.

Finger Extension

Strengthen each finger by gently pressing the palm flat on a table. This helps prevent loss of movement in the fingers. (See Figure 5.20.)

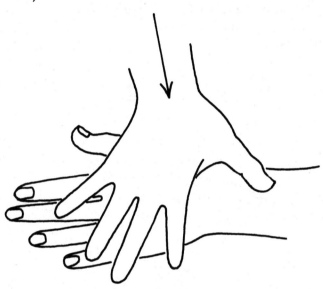

Figure 5.20.   A finger extension exercise.

Thumb and Finger Touch

This is a simple exercise that accomplishes the very important function of grasp and pinch in the finger and hand. (See Figure 5.21.)

Try to form the letter O with your thumb and each finger on the hand. After you make the O, straighten the fingers and touch the next finger. Make an O and then straighten. Be sure the thumb rounds into a good O.

Repeat this, gradually increasing up to 5, then 10 repetitions. Repeat this exercise two times each day.

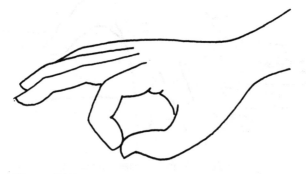

Figure 5.21.　A thumb and finger touch exercise.

Finger Abduction and Adduction

Spread the fingers as widely apart as possible. (See Figure 5.22.) Then close them together as tightly as possible. Hold for a count of 6. Repeat twice daily, gradually increasing to 20 repetitions each session.

Place your hand flat on a table. Pick up and move each finger individually toward the thumb. (See Figure 5.23.) This will help prevent drifting of the fingers toward the little finger side of the hand.

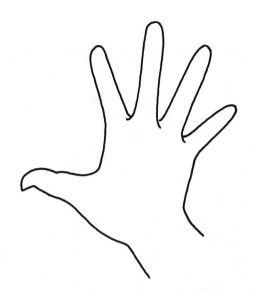

Figure 5.22. A finger abduction and adduction exercise.

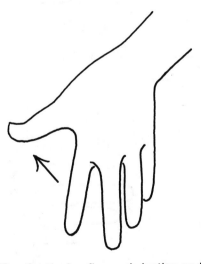

Figure 5.23. Continuing finger abduction and adduction.

Thumb

   Place your hand flat on a table, with palm facing up. (See Figure 5.24.)

1. Push the thumb away from the hand.
2. Bring the thumb toward the hand.
3. Lift the thumb off the table.
4. Bend the thumb down and repeat the sequence 20 times twice daily.

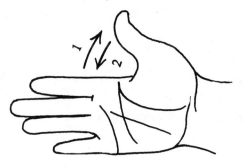

3

4

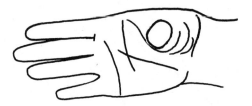

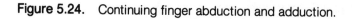

Figure 5.24.   Continuing finger abduction and adduction.

Hip Exercises

Hip Flexion

This is a good exercise to do before you get out of bed in the morning to help you limber up for the day. It also stretches the hips, the lower back, and the knees. These exercises can be done on the bed or on the floor if you are able. (See Figure 5.25.)

Bend each knee to the chest, one at a time. If assistance is needed, put hands under a knee and help it bend to the chest. Repeat this, alternating knees. Do 5, then 10, then 20 repetitions two or three times a day if possible.

Now pull both knees to your chest at the same time and hold for 6 seconds. Gently rock from side to side while holding the knees. Repeat this exercise, increasing gradually to 5, then 10, then 20 repetitions two or three sessions a day if possible.

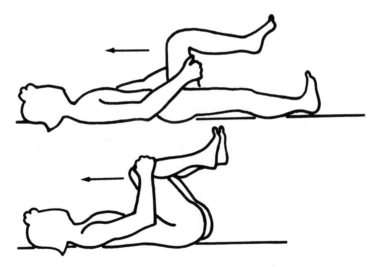

Figure 5.25. A hip flexion exercise.

Hip Abduction

This exercise to improve the mobility of the hips is done lying on your bed or on the floor, whichever is the most comfortable for you. (See Figure 5.26.)

Lie on your back. Bend one leg so that your knee is straight up and pointed to the ceiling. Slide the leg out toward the side and then return. Repeat with the opposite leg. Gradually increase to 5, then 10, then 20 repetitions two or three times a day if possible.

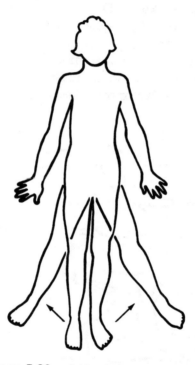

Figure 5.26. A hip abduction exercise.

Hip Extension

The position for this exercise is lying on your stomach. This can be done on the bed or floor if you are able.

A pillow placed under the stomach may make lying on the floor more comfortable.

With the knee straight, raise the thigh straight up behind you, lifting it off the floor. (See Figure 5.27.) If you lift too far, you will rotate your pelvis and will not get the desired movement. Now lift the other thigh. When you lift your thigh slightly off the floor, try counting six seconds while you hold the motion. This is an isometric exercise to help build muscle strength. You may experience some cramping when you do this because your muscles are working hard to accomplish this motion. Try massaging the muscle. If it persists, talk to your physician or physical therapist.

Repeat this motion and gradually increase up to 5, then 10 repetitions if you can. Repeat this two times daily if possible.

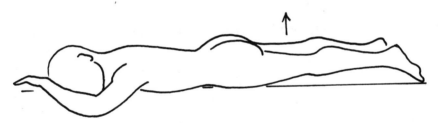

Figure 5.27.   A hip extension exercise.

Hip Rotation

To do this exercise, lie on your bed or on the floor. This exercise may seem like a foot exercise but it actually rotates your hips when you keep your legs straight. (See Figure 5.28.)

Lie on your back. Turn your knees in and touch your toes together. Now turn your knees out.

Repeat this exercise, gradually increasing up to 5, then 10, then 20 repetitions each session. Repeat this exercise two times daily.

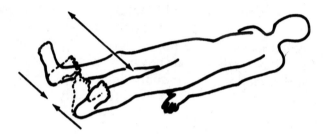

Figure 5.28.   A hip rotation exercise.

Knee and Leg Exercises

Knee Extension

Sit in a chair and support your foot on a table or chair that is of comfortable height. This is a two-part exercise. (See Figure 5.29.)

By simply straightening your leg, you are maintaining knee flexibility. Make it as straight as you can tolerate and hold at that point.

Now, add an isometric strengthening exercise. Try pulling your toes up so the back of the leg is stretched. Tighten your knee cap by pushing the knee down a little and hold the contraction. You will notice wrinkles in the knee cap and the muscles in the thigh tighten. Hold that contraction for six seconds, relax, and repeat. This exercise is especially important for knee stability and standing support. It is called quadriceps muscle (quad) setting. (See Figure 5.30.)

This is a very important exercise to maintain knee strength. Begin gradually and work up to 12 repetitions at one time. Repeat this two or three times a day. This exercise can be done while you relax in a chair watching television or at work for a change of position and release of tension.

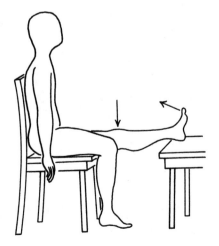

Figure 5.29.   A knee extension exercise.

Quad Setting (Quadriceps Muscle Setting)

Figure 5.30 illustrates pushing the knee down and tightening the kneecap. Hold this position for six counts.

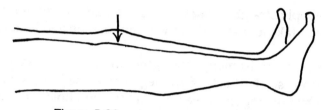

Figure 5.30. A quad setting exercise.

Straight Leg Raise

This exercise helps strengthen the large muscles in the front of the thigh (the quadriceps) that are a major support for the knee. It also strengthens the muscles of the abdomen and improves the flexibility of the legs. Lie on your bed or on the floor, whichever is more comfortable for you.

Lie flat on your back. To protect your back during this exercise, you may hug one leg to your chest or simply bend the knee and hip, and rest the foot on the bed. (See Figure 5.31 for both positions.) Choose the position most comfortable for you. Now raise the other leg straight up slowly as far as you can, trying to keep the abdomen in and maintaining the back firmly against the floor or bed as in the pelvic tilt-flat back position. When your back begins to arch, stop the raised leg at that point. Hold the position for 6 seconds. Bend and lower the leg and repeat the exercise. Now do the same for the other leg.

Repeat this exercise, gradually increasing up to 5, then 10, then up to 20 repetitions. If your back hurts or if you have pain in your leg, talk to your physician or physical therapist before you continue.

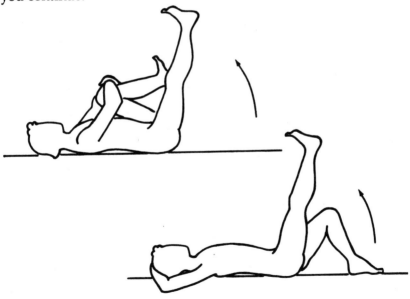

Figure 5.31.   A straight leg raise exercise.

Knee Flexion

This exercise can be done on your bed or on the floor, whichever is more comfortable. Lying on your stomach, bend your knee, moving your ankle toward your back as far as you can, then straighten your knee again. Repeat this, alternating legs. Gradually increase to 5, then 10, then 20 repetitions twice each day. (See Figure 5.32.)

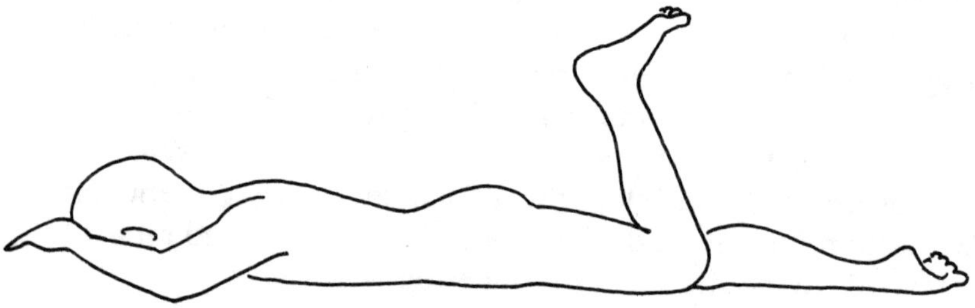

Figure 5.32.   A knee flexion exercise.

Ankle and Feet Exercises

Ankles and Feet

These exercises increase the flexibility and strength in the ankles and feet. The best position for these exercises is sitting in a chair with the feet flat on the floor. (See Figure 5.33.)

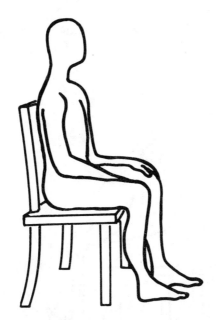

Figure 5.33.   Position for ankle and feet exercises.

1. Raise your toes as high as you can while keeping your heel on the floor. (See Figure 5.34.) Keep your toes down and lift your heels as high as possible.
2. Lift the inside of each foot and roll the weight over on the outside of the foot. Keep your toes curled down, if possible. The soles of your feet should be turned in facing each other. (See Figure 5.35.)
3. Rotate the ankle in a circle, curling toes up and down and around in a circle. (See Figure 5.36.)

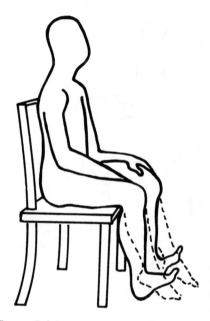

Figure 5.34.　An ankle and feet exercise.

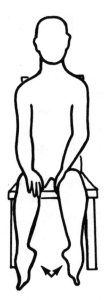

Figure 5.35. An ankle and feet exercise.

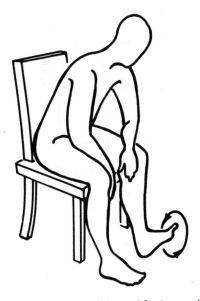

Figure 5.36. An ankle and feet exercise.

Back Exercises

Cheek to Cheek

This is a fun exercise because you can do it anywhere, anytime, and practically in any position. This exercise strengthens the muscles of the buttocks that help support the back and the legs. When sitting, you will actually raise up out of the chair because of the contraction of the muscle groups in the buttocks. (See Figure 5.37.)

Press your buttocks together and hold for a 6-second count. Relax and repeat. Gradually increase up to 5, then 10, then 20 repetitions. Repeat two times daily.

This exercise can be done frequently during the day as tolerated wherever you may be.

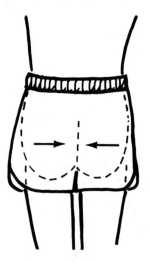

Figure 5.37.　A cheek to cheek exercise.

Pelvic Tilt

This is one of the best exercises you can do to strengthen your abdominal muscles which in turn help support your back. This exercise will also help tone your stomach muscles. Do this exercise lying in bed or on the floor, whichever is more comfortable. (See Figure 5.38.)

Relax and raise your arms above your head. Keep your knees bent. Now comes the tricky part. Tighten the muscles of your lower abdomen and your buttocks at the same time to flatten your back against the floor or bed. This is the flat back position that you now hold for a 6-second count. Now relax and repeat.

This is sometimes a difficult exercise to understand. If you have trouble, contact your physical therapist or physician and have them demonstrate the exercise.

Repeat this exercise 2 or 3 times to start and work gradually to 5, then 10, then 20 repetitions.

This exercise can also be done standing up or sitting in a chair but probably requires some demonstration by a physical therapist for these positions.

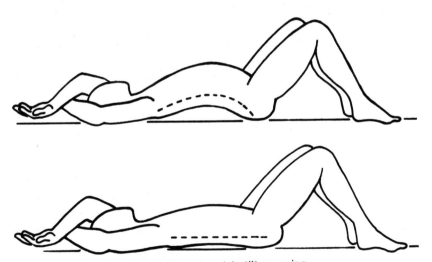

Figure 5.38.   A pelvic tilt exercise.

Bridging

This exercise is done lying in bed or on the floor. It strengthens the muscles in the back. (See Figure 5.39.)

Lie on the floor and bend (flex) your hips and knees. Now lift your hips and buttocks off the bed or floor 4 to 6 inches, forcing the small of the back out flat; and tighten the buttock and hip muscles to maintain this position. Hold this position for a count of six seconds. Now, relax and lower your hips and buttocks to the floor. Repeat.

Repeat this exercise, gradually increasing up to 5, then 10, then 20 repetitions as tolerated. Do this twice daily if possible.

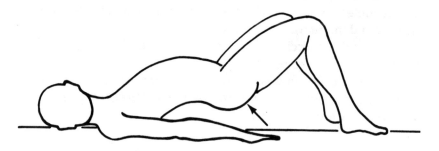

Figure 5.39.   A bridging exercise.

Partial Sit-Up

This is one of the more vigorous exercises. It is an exercise to build abdominal strength which in turn better supports the back. (See Figure 5.40.)

To do this exercise, lie on your bed or on the floor, whichever is more comfortable.

Lie on your back with your knees bent. The goal of this exercise is to raise your head and shoulder blades off the floor or bed. Now hold that position for a 6-second count. Slowly return to the beginning position of lying on your back. Repeat.

Start this exercise slowly with 1 or 2 repetitions until your body adjusts to the exercise. Gradually increase to 5, then 10 repetitions. Be sure to do all strengthening exercises and count 6 seconds out loud as it is very important that you breathe properly while holding the position. By counting out loud, you will breathe properly. If you experience shortness of breath, stop and talk to your doctor or physical therapist.

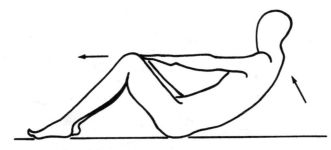

Figure 5.40.   A partial sit-up exercise.

Back Extension

This exercise for strengthening the back muscles is for lying on your bed or on the floor in a prone (stomach down) position (See Figure 5.41). A pillow may be used under the stomach to help make this position more comfortable.

Raise your head, arms, and legs off the floor. Do not bend your knees. This must be done with your body straight in extension. Hold for several seconds while you count out loud. Relax and repeat.

Gradually increase this exercise up to 5, then 10 repetitions. If you experience discomfort, check with your physician or physical therapist before you continue.

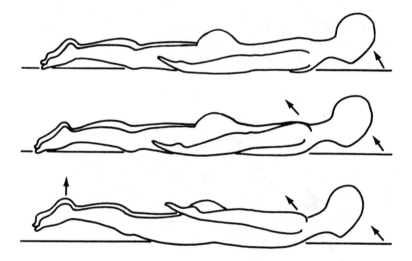

Figure 5.41.   A back extension exercise.

Cat Camel

Do not do this exercise for strengthening the back muscles if you have very painful knees, ankles, or hands. It places pressure on these areas. (See Figure 5.42.)

The position for this exercise is a crawling position. Hands must be directly under your shoulders. Take a deep breath and arch your back as a frightened cat does, lowering your head. Hold that position while you count the 6 seconds out loud. Now exhale and drop the arched back slowly, raising your head.

Start this exercise slowly with one or two repetitions. Increase up to 5 and then 10 repetitions if possible.

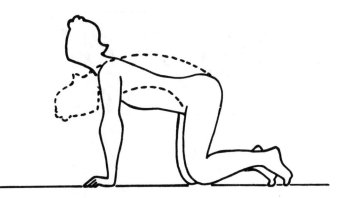

Figure 5.42. A cat camel exercise.

Wall Push

This exercise is good for persons with arthritis in the back, especially ankylosing spondylitis, because it encourages the body extension positions.

Stand spread eagle against a solid wall. Now arch your back inward slowly.

Repeat this exercise and gradually increase repetitions from 1 to 5 or more. This exercise is fun because you can do it any time you feel you need a good body stretch. Repeat two times daily. (See Figure 5.43.)

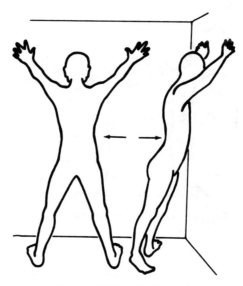

Figure 5.43. Wall push.

Back Flexibility

Lie on your back on the floor with knees bent and feet flat on the floor. Raise hands toward the ceiling. Now move arms and turn the head to the right, while the knees move to the left. Reverse the above, then repeat. Gradually increase up to 5 and then 10 repetitions daily. (See Figure 5.44.)

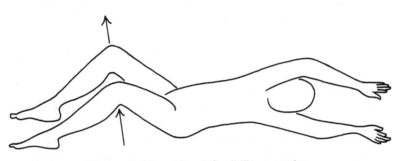

Figure 5.44.   A back flexibility exercise.

Bicycling

Lying on your back, move your feet and legs in the air as if you were riding a bicycle. Count to 6, and relax. Repeat, then gradually increase to 5 and then 10 repetitions once or twice daily if tolerated. (See Figure 5.45.)

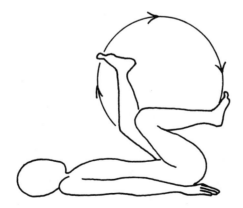

Figure 5.45.   A bicycling exercise.

Chest and Posture Exercises

Deep Breathing

This exercise improves the movement of the chest and helps your posture. This exercise is performed in the rest position with your hands comfortably placed behind your head. You will also do a good shoulder rotation exercise by placing your hands behind your head. This position allows your rib cage and chest to expand fully. Bend your knees to protect your back. (See Figure 5.46.)

Once you are in this comfortable position, breathe deeply and raise your chest while filling your lungs completely. Hold for about two seconds and then exhale by drawing your upper abdomen in. Take the next breath against the uplifted chest. This may be a difficult exercise to understand without a demonstration. Contact your physical therapist or physician for assistance.

Begin this exercise slowly and gradually increase the repetitions from 5 to 10, then up to 20.

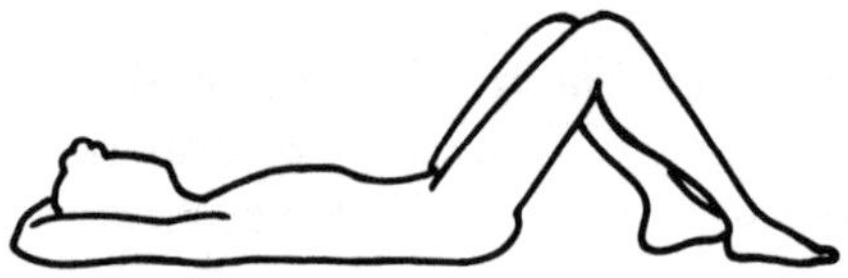

Figure 5.46.   A deep breathing exercise.

Wing Back

This is another exercise that is good for people with arthritis in the back because it encourages the bending of the arms and body backwards. (See Figure 5.47.)

This exercise is done in a relaxed standing position. Lift your elbows to shoulder height with arms bent. Now straighten arms backwards. Hold.

Repeat this exercise and gradually increase the repetitions. Start with 5 and work up to 10, then 20 as tolerated. Repeat the exercise two times daily.

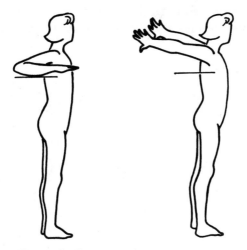

Figure 5.47.   A wing back exercise.

Arm Swing

The object of these exercises is to emphasize extension of the back and neck and increased expansion of the chest. All of these motions are important for people with arthritis in the back, especially ankylosing spondylitis. Posture is important when doing these exercises. Stand comfortably with your knees, back, and shoulders slightly relaxed. (See Figure 5.48.)

Start with your hands down and crossed in front of you. Swing them slowly up and out over the head, reaching back as far as you can. When your arms are up take a deep breath. When you lower your arms exhale. Repeat.

Repeat this exercise, gradually increasing up to 5, then 10 repetitions. This exercise should be repeated two times daily.

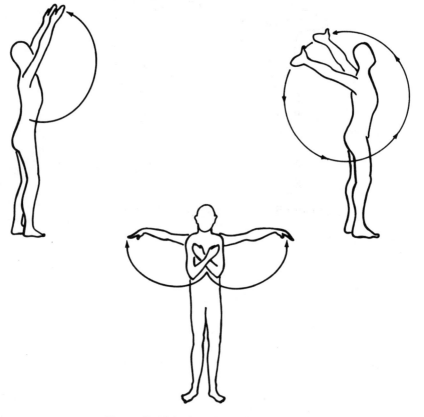

Figure 5.48. An arm swing exercise.

Diagonal Arm Swing

Start with both arms out to the side at hip height. Move diagonally across your body and upward over your head. Twisting the trunk, turn the head to watch the hands, inhale on the upswing and exhale on the downswing. Reverse and do the other side. Repeat. Gradually increase up to 5, then 10 repetitions daily. (See Figure 5.49.)

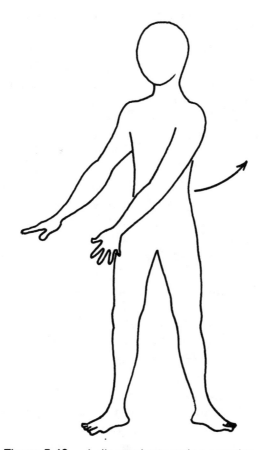

Figure 5.49. A diagonal arm swing exercise.

Strengthening Exercises

When the above exercises can be easily performed up to 20 or more repetitions without pain or other discomfort, it may be possible to begin a more aggressive type of exercise to try to gain more muscle strength. Before you attempt this, discuss it with your physician or physical therapist to be sure that it is safe for you.

Two easy ways to begin to build more muscle strength are the use of isometric exercises and light weights.

Isometric exercises use muscle contractions without joint movement. This works well in many people with arthritis since joint movement may be painful, especially at first. The resistance should be very light at first, then very gradually increased as pain allows and as strength increases.

Figures 5.50 to 5.55 are a few examples of isometric exercises using a rubber or elastic band or with the hands as resistance.

Light hand or ankle weights may sometimes be used to strengthen muscles. The usual exercises as described are performed with the addition of 1 or 2 pound weights on the ankles, feet, arms, or hands. Weights must be very light, such as 1 or 2 pounds, to avoid adding excess stress to the joints being exercised.

The light weights can be strapped to the hand, wrist, or ankle. If no weights are available, we suggest using canned goods by holding them in the hands to exercise the shoulders and elbows as tolerated. A sock filled with sand and with the top tied can be used as a weight for the wrist or ankle in some cases. (See Figure 5.56.)

Remember, it is more important to begin an exercise program gradually and safely than to do a large amount of exercise quickly. Your exercise program should be part of a long-term plan using the basic treatment program for arthritis. Stay with it, and you'll be surprised how quickly you can do many more exercises than you expected. After a few weeks to months you will begin to see more flexibility and more strength, and you will have less pain in the joints. This will allow much more activity. You will be able to do the things you could not do earlier because of pain and stiffness.

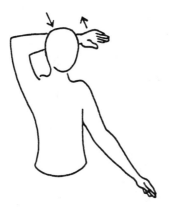

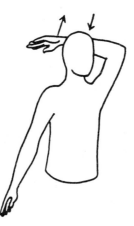

Figure 5.50. Isometric exercises for the neck.

Isometric Exercises for the Neck

1. With one hand or forearm placed on the forehead, try to look downward with the head while at the same time resisting this movement with the hand or forearm .
Hold for 5 to 6 seconds. Breathe. Then repeat. Do one, then two, then gradually increase up to 5, then 10 times twice each day.

2. Now with the hand or forearm on the *back* of the head, try to look upward while resisting the movement with the hand or forearm as shown in Figure 5.50. Hold for 5 to 6 seconds. Breathe. Then repeat. Do one, then 2, then gradually increase up to 5, then 10 times twice each day.

Isometric Exercises for the Shoulders

1. Using a rubber or elastic band (your physician or physical therapist can supply this) pull both arms out towards the side of the body as shown. When the band is tight, giving resistance, hold in that position for 5 to 6 seconds. (See Figure 5.51.)

2. Pull one arm upward and the opposite arm downward. When the band is tight, giving resistance, hold in that position for 5 to 6 seconds.

3. With one arm behind the back and the other arm behind the head, pull upward and downward as shown until the band is tight, giving resistance. Hold for 5 to 6 seconds.

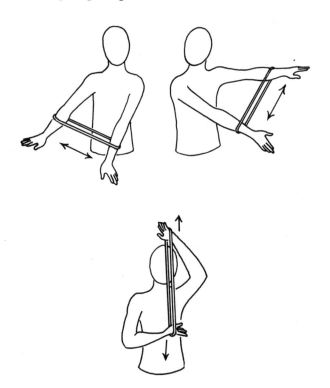

Figure 5.51. Isometric exercises for the shoulders.

Isometric Exercises for the Elbows

With the elbows bent and the elastic band placed around the forearms, try to bend one elbow toward your chest while straightening the other elbow out. (See Figures 5.52 and 5.53.) Hold for 5 to 6 seconds when the band becomes tight. The band should be 12 to 18 inches in length. Your physical therapist or physician can help if you have questions about these exercises.

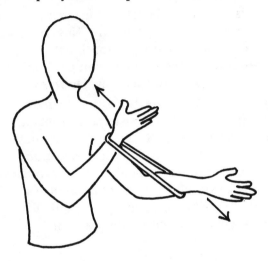

Figure 5.52.   An isometric exercise for the elbows.

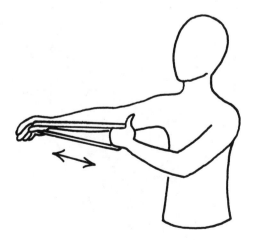

Figure 5.53.   An isometric exercise for the elbows.

Isometric Exercises for the Wrist and Fingers

1. With your hands resting on a table, place one hand on top of the hand on the table. Then the bottom hand tries to lift upward while the hand on top presses down to give resistance. (See Figure 5.54.) Hold for 5 to 6 seconds. Repeat once, then twice, then gradually increase up to 10 times twice each day. Do this for both hands.

2. With hands resting on the table, place one hand on the back of the fingers. Now try to lift the fingers upwards while pressing downward with the top hand. Hold 5 to 6 seconds. Repeat once, then twice, then gradually increase up to 5 then 10 times twice each day. Do this for both hands.

3. With your hands on the table, try to move each finger towards the thumb but resist the movement by pushing with the index finger of the *other* hand as shown. Hold 5 to 6 seconds. Repeat once, then twice, then gradually increase up to 5 then 10 times twice daily. Do this for each finger on both hands. Start with very light resistance at first to avoid pain in the fingers and hands, then gradually increase the resistance as you can without more pain.

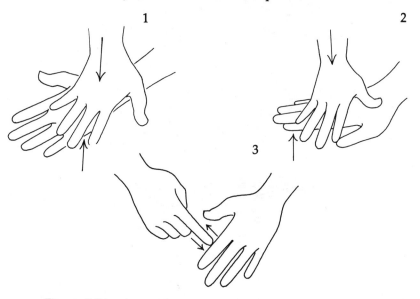

Figure 5.54. Isometric exercises for the wrist and fingers.

Isometric Exercises for the Hips

1. Sitting in a chair with the hands on your outer thighs, pull your legs apart while both hands push inward. (See Figure 5.55.) This gives resistance to the movement. Hold 5 to 6 seconds. Do once, then twice, and gradually increase as you can up to 10 times twice daily.

   This exercise can also be done with the hands on the *inside* of the thighs. The legs then pull *together* while the hands push *outward*.

2. Place the elastic band above the ankles. Lying face down on the bed or floor, raise one leg upward while the other leg remains on the bed or floor. Hold for 5 to 6 seconds. Repeat once, then twice and gradually increase up to 10 times twice daily.

3. Raise up on the toes and hold this position for 5 to 6 seconds. (See Figure 5.55(3).) Repeat once, then twice, then gradually increase up to 10 times twice daily. This can help strengthen the ankles and the calf muscles.

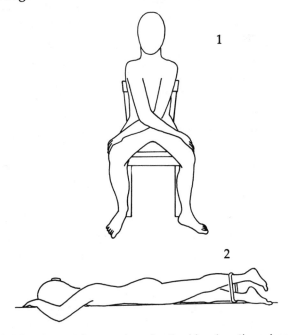

1

2

Figure 5.55.   Isometric exercises for the hips (continued on page 138).

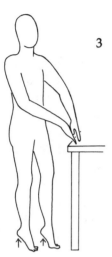

3

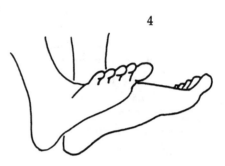

4

Figure 5.55. (continued)

Examples of Exercises Using Light Weights

1. With the weight strapped around the wrist, raise the arm upward towards the head and back to the side of the body. Repeat once, then twice, then gradually increase up to 10 times twice daily.

2. Arm circles can be done with the weights around the wrist. Start with a small circle, gradually increasing the size of the circle. Repeat once, then twice, then gradually increase up to 10 times twice each day if possible. Don't overdo this exercise at first, and remember to use light weights of only 1 pound at first.

3. Lying on the bed, slide one leg out to the side and back to the middle with the weight strapped just above the ankle. Do this for both legs. Repeat once, then twice, then gradually increase up to 10 times twice each day as you can comfortably do without pain.

4. Sitting in a chair, with the weight strapped at the ankle, straighten the knee out and lower back down to the floor. Be sure to go only as far as is comfortable, and use only light weights of 1 pound. Repeat once, then twice, and then gradually increase up to 5 or 10 times twice daily if you can do this without pain. (See Figure 5.56.)

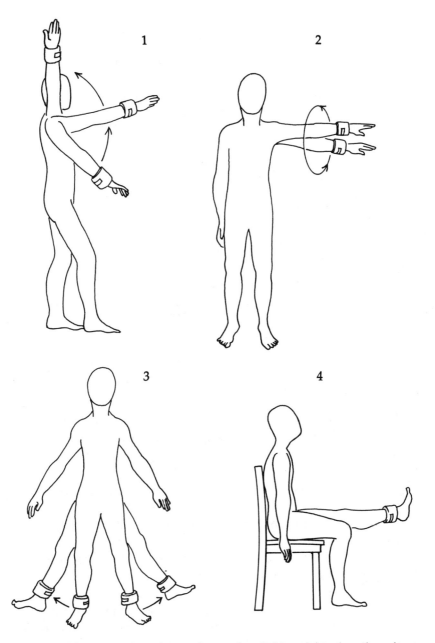

Figure 5.56 Examples of exercises using light weights (continued on page 140).

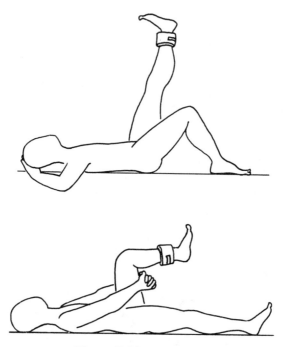

Figure 5.56 (continued)

As we mentioned previously, the use of moist heat along with the exercises makes them easier and less painful. Once you are able to tolerate a regular program, these exercises will be even more effective in producing flexible joints and stronger muscles.

If your arthritis is severe or if you are not used to exercises, don't allow yourself to avoid the moist heat and exercises. Remember, there is no limit on exercises by age. It may be necessary for you to begin your heat and exercise program with the help of regular visits to a physical therapist. Then as you improve, you can manage the program at home with visits to the therapist as needed.

When your arthritis improves, don't stop the exercise program. It can be adjusted for more convenience, but should be continued indefinitely for maximum strength and mobility.

CHAPTER SIX

Surgery and Other Available Treatment

If the basic treatment plan is not effective or gives only partial relief, alternative treatments are available. Depending on the type of arthritis you have, some treatments are more effective than others.

When to Consider Surgery

Surgery is an option when the following conditions exist:

1. There is *severe pain* or *severe loss of use* of a joint, and
2. The *basic treatment plan* is not enough.

As with any treatment, your overall health must be a consideration before surgery becomes an option. Your physician will help you decide if your health is good enough to consider surgery. Age alone does not usually prevent surgery in arthritis. Rather, overall health considerations must be taken into account. Since there are some risks in every surgery, it is best to understand what the benefits and the risks of the operation may be. You can then make a good decision. Good results in arthritis *depend strongly* on hard work in physical therapy and exercise *after* surgery.

We'll discuss some of the instances in which surgery can prove helpful.

Surgery for Osteoarthritis

In osteoarthritis when the basic treatment plan has not provided adequate improvement in pain, it is appropriate to look at other means of treatment. Also, when there is more and more loss of use of a joint or deformities are present, surgery is a good option to consider. As discussed, surgery *may not* always be possible because of the risk of other medical problems. Each person is different, and the benefits of surgery are decided on an individual basis.

Since osteoarthritis often only affects one or two joints severely, the relief given by surgery may allow much improvement and more activity. The hips and the knees are the most common joints considered for surgery in osteoarthritis. Surgery in osteoarthritis of other joints is less common but available. This includes the shoulder, elbow, ankle, wrist, and fingers. Surgery for osteoarthritis in the neck or lower back is usually done only when the arthritis has resulted in pressure on a nerve root in the cervical or lumbar spine.

Total Joint Replacement

Total joint replacement (total joint arthroplasty) is now widely available in most medical centers. Where indicated in persons having osteoarthritis, total joint replacement of hips and knees offers relief of pain as well as greatly increased mobility. An orthopedic surgeon performs the replacement surgery and can tell you what the chances are for improvement in pain and use of the joint in your particular situation.

In addition to the hip and knee, total joint replacement for the shoulder has been used with excellent results in some centers. There is usually good relief of shoulder pain and improvement in use of the shoulder. This newer surgery is not as widely available as total hip or knee replacement since fewer orthopedic surgeons have experience with the operation. Replacement of other joints is available in some medical centers.

Arthroscopy

In *arthroscopy,* the joint is viewed directly by a light inserted through a small incision and damaged cartilage or other problems can then be corrected. The recovery time is usually much faster than with other surgery or total replacement surgery. Arthroscopy is used less often in severe cases of osteoarthritis because the cartilage is either absent or already too severely damaged to repair.

Other Procedures

Procedures used less often since total joint replacement has been available are *osteotomy* and *fusion. Osteotomy* is the procedure used when bones of the joint are straightened and aligned so that weight bearing is more effective again. This is done mainly in the knee and often gives good pain relief. It is thought by many orthopedic surgeons to be a way to provide relief for a few years and to delay total knee replacement. Improvement may last for 5 to 9 years depending on the situation. Total knee replacement can still be done at a later time. Your orthopedic surgeon can tell you if this would be a good idea in your own situation.

Another surgery for joints is *fusion, or arthrodesis.* The joint is fused together so no movement is possible. This results in relief of pain but loss of flexibility of the joint. It is used in the ankle with good results, but is not used in the knee or hip when total joint replacement is available and preferable.

Surgery for Bursitis and Tendinitis

In bursitis and tendinitis, surgery is less often needed for treatment. However, if there is not a good response and activity is still quite limited after basic treatment, an evaluation by an orthopedic surgeon would be helpful. There may be another

Total joint replacement
Arthroscopy
Osteotomy
Fusion

Figure 6.1.   Most common types of surgery in osteoarthritis.

problem aggravating the bursitis or tendinitis that may be treatable. For example, bursitis or tendinitis in a shoulder may not respond to treatment because there may be a tear in the tendon or other tissues that support the shoulder. In such a case, surgery may give very effective relief. Some forms of tendinitis and bursitis may benefit from surgery if they do not respond to medical treatment.

Surgery is sometimes needed when a tendon and its surrounding sheath in the palm of the hand are inflamed, called *"trigger finger."* A finger may "catch" in a bent position when it is moved and cause pain when it is straightened. This can be painful and limit the use of the finger in a handgrip and other activities. A local injection often gives relief. When the injection is not effective, surgery can correct the problem.

Treatment for Fibrositis (Fibromyalgia)

In fibrositis cases, surgery is not helpful. However, if fibrositis does not respond to the basic treatment plan then one of a group of medications may give relief.

This other group of medications has been used for other medical problems for many years. Some of the most common have also been used as anti-depressants. In lower doses than usually needed for depression, these medications may have some anti-inflammatory effect and control pain in fibrositis.

As shown in Table 6.1, there are several different medications in this group. It is usually necessary to try a few different ones to find the medication most effective for you. The response

Table 6.1
Some Medications Used in Fibrositis (Fibromyalgia)

Trade Name	Generic Name
Elavil	Amitriptyline
Tofranil	Imipramine
Flexeril (also used a muscle relaxant, not used as anti-depressant)	Cyclobenzaprine
Sinequan	Doxepin

may be excellent with relief from pain and stiffness, improved activity, and improved sleep pattern at night. The response is usually seen over a period of several weeks.

When one of these medications is combined with an effective anti-inflammatory drug, most persons gain control of the pain, stiffness, and loss of activity. Because it takes weeks to months to find the correct combination for each person, it can be very frustrating to both patient and physician. But the relief of severely limiting pain, stiffness, and fatigue of fibrositis is worth the time and effort.

Since the doses of these medications used are usually lower than when used for depression, the side effects are generally less. The most common side effects are mouth dryness, constipation, dizziness, palpitations (rapid or forceful heart beat), or a calming (sedating) effect. At higher doses or in older persons, difficulty in urination or blurred vision can result. Persons with glaucoma or prostate problems should take these medications with special caution. In some people, these medications produce weakness or fatigue. Fluid retention or cardiac problems can be aggravated, or tremors may occur, but usually at higher doses than used in fibrositis. In addition, individual allergic reactions can happen as with any drug.

No blood tests are routinely needed when these medications are taken in low doses. If any new problems or side effects develop, you should contact your physician to be sure the problem is not due to the medication.

If improvement from fibrositis is still not adequate, then some other pain control techniques are needed. The management of chronic pain is discussed in Chapter 8.

Surgery for Rheumatoid Arthritis

If the basic treatment plan for rheumatoid arthritis combined with a suppressive drug as outlined in Chapter 4 does not give enough improvement then surgery may be a consideration.

The procedures available include removal of the swollen, thickened lining of the joint (called *synovectomy*). This is a consideration when other treatment does not control the arthritis. It is usually done before there is a lot of destruction in the joint itself. In the wrist, it may help prevent damage to the tendons which control the use of the fingers. This treatment might prevent later surgery by prevention of a tendon rupture which causes loss of movement in a finger.

This procedure may also be used in the knee. It does not stop the arthritis, but gives improvement that may last a few years. After an average of about five years, there is often a return of the arthritis in the knee. *Arthroscopy,* in which there is direct examination of the lining of the joint, can also be used to perform synovectomy in the knee, although there is some controversy as to its overall effectiveness.

Surgery may also be helpful in a problem caused by arthritis in the wrist. Swelling may cause pressure on a nerve (median nerve) as it passes through the wrist near the palm of the hand. This causes numbness, tingling, and at times weakness in the fingers and is called *carpal tunnel syndrome.* It is a common problem in rheumatoid arthritis as well as other types of arthritis or may happen alone. If there is no response to a basic treatment plan, then surgery may be needed to release the pressure on the nerve. This is usually done on an outpatient basis.

Total joint replacement (total joint arthroplasty) is also used in rheumatoid arthritis when the pain in a joint cannot be controlled or if there is severe damage to the joint. It is used when there is continued loss of use of a joint and severe damage to the joint by the arthritis. Extreme deformities and loss of use of the joint may also be corrected by total joint replacement.

Total hip or knee replacements usually give good relief of pain with improvement in mobility and use of the joint. Removal of the most severe pain may lead to an overall improvement. This may allow other medical treatment to control the rest of the joints involved.

Your physician and your orthopedic surgeon can guide you if surgery is needed to treat your rheumatoid arthritis. Most

Synovectomy
Arthroscopy
Total joint replacement (total joint arthroplasty)

Figure 6.2.   Common types of surgery in rheumatoid arthritis.

patients do not need surgery. But when the proper operation is chosen at the proper time, you can expect a high chance of relief of pain and improvement in function.

Nonsurgical Treatment for Systemic Lupus Erythematosus

In systemic lupus erythematosus (SLE or lupus), many patients do well if they maintain the basic treatment plan discussed in Chapter 4. A program of heat and exercises, nonsteroid anti-inflammatory drugs, and use of the lowest possible dose of one of the cortisone derivatives when necessary usually allows good control of the disease.

In some cases, the basic treatment program for lupus will not be enough. When internal organ involvement is severe enough, other suppressive medications may be needed to gain control of the disease. Drugs in this group of medications attempt to suppress the activity of lupus. This may help control the disease without cortisone derivatives. Or, using one of these drugs may permit the reduction of the dose of a cortisone derivative, usually prednisone. The side effects of higher doses of cortisone derivatives may then be minimized while succeeding in controlling the disease.

Surgery for Lupus

Surgery in lupus is used mainly for complications of the disease. One of the more common types of arthritis surgery is needed when there is collapse of a portion of a bone in the shoulder or hip. This condition (called ischemic necrosis) can cause severe pain in addition to that present due to arthritis.

Nonsurgical Treatment for Juvenile Rheumatoid Arthritis

The basic treatment program in Chapter 4 is usually effective in juvenile rheumatoid arthritis; many children show improvement so that signs and feelings of the arthritis become minimized or a remission occurs.

However, in some cases, the arthritis may continue to be limiting or may be severe enough to require a cortisone derivative such as prednisone for control. A second medication from the suppressive group of drugs used in adult rheumatoid arthritis may allow better control of the arthritis. It may allow the cortisone derivative to be stopped, or at least used in the lowest possible dose.

In these younger patients, the dosage and side effects of any medication must be carefully assessed. Some of the suppressive drugs have been used more widely in children than others. When parents and physician monitor the medication and its effects then one of these can usually be given safely to allow better control of the disease.

Surgery for Juvenile Rheumatoid Arthritis

Surgery is sometimes used in juvenile rheumatoid arthritis although much less often than in adults. Removal of the lining of the joint (synovectomy) is done at times in older children when there is only one joint involved.

Total joint replacement is now considered at younger ages than in earlier years, but there is concern over how long the new joint will last. Each situation is unique and must be treated differently.

Surgery can also be used to release tightened muscles and tendons to allow more movement. In some cases, fusion of a joint (arthrodesis) can help a severe deformity and allow more activity.

To be successful, parent and child must be able to cooperate and help in the recovery and rehabilitation needed after surgery.

Treatment for Psoriatic Arthritis

The basic treatment program for psoriatic arthritis is often successful in controlling the pain, stiffness, and swelling. When heat, exercises and nonsteroid anti-inflammatory drugs are not enough for good control, then some of the suppressive drugs used to control severe rheumatoid arthritis may be helpful. Methotrexate and gold are the most commonly used of this group of medications in psoriatic arthritis. Their use is usually similar to use in rheumatoid arthritis.

Surgery may be used for joints severely affected by psoriatic arthritis as in rheumatoid arthritis, including total joint replacement.

Surgery for Ankylosing Spondylitis

Surgery may be useful in cases of ankylosing spondylitis. It is most commonly needed when there is severe hip involvement with total joint replacement. Other situations that may require surgery are those in which there is pressure on a nerve as it exits the spine or other complications of the arthritis involving the spine.

Surgery for Arthritis of the Foot

When the basic treatment program, proper shoes, and other foot care is not enough, surgery may be helpful. You should be aware of the plans of the surgeon, including a discussion of the alternative methods of treatment as well as the possible risks or possibilities of less than desirable results. Don't hesitate to ask questions if you don't understand everything clearly.

In early arthritis, surgery may release tightened tendons around the diseased joint to improve or delay deformity. These may not be permanent answers to the problems that can recur later.

Joint replacements in the foot are available, although these carry risks that may increase in older patients. Loosening of the artificial joint and infection can occur.

Removal of part of a joint or bone in the toes can give improvement in pain and deformity. At times, these procedures can give the disabled some level of walking they had not thought possible.

Many procedures can be done under local anesthesia allowing people to walk limited distances immediately after surgery in special casts or surgical shoes. Extensive surgery can allow the patient immediate mobility on crutches when performed on one foot at a time. When hospital treatment is required, the patient usually leaves without an overnight stay.

Don't hesitate to ask questions or to seek a second opinion until you are comfortable that you have all the needed facts to make the correct decision about surgery for your arthritis.

CHAPTER SEVEN

Diets and
Nonstandard Treatment

The causes and cures for most kinds of arthritis are not known. This means that many persons, especially those who don't get proper treatment, suffer for months or even years. Any disease that does not have a well-defined cure and cause becomes the subject of folk cures and remedies. People with arthritis find that every well-meaning friend, neighbor, and relative seem ready to offer them the solution or cure.

Diet and Arthritis—New Facts, Old Fiction

Many people with arthritis wonder about the importance of diet in the treatment of arthritis. Diet can be important in different ways for many of the more than 100 types of arthritis. For example, diet was known to be important in gout several hundred years ago. In gout, there is a high level of uric acid in the blood (see page 30). The uric acid level may increase if the diet is very rich in organ meats (liver, kidney, brain), and other high protein foods.

Gout became known as a badge of the wealthy, because they could afford the diet that produced gout. Medieval cookbooks commonly showed 5 or 6 courses in one meal containing meats and other high protein foods!

151

Alcohol Increases Blood Uric Acid Level

The average diet today is not the major cause of gout since it contains less of the foods that produce high uric acid levels. The most common way in which diet affects gout today is by alcohol consumption. Large amounts of alcohol, especially over a short time (such as a "party weekend"), can cause an increase in the blood uric acid level and result in an attack of gout. Today's medicines are so effective that diet is not a major limitation otherwise in gout.

Elimination of Foods

The role of diet in other types of arthritis is more controversial. Many patients with osteoarthritis and rheumatoid arthritis complain that certain foods seem to cause a worsening or flare up of their arthritis. This has led to many diet remedies for arthritis by elimination of foods. Some feel their arthritis worsens when they eat tomato products, citrus products, red meats, or other food items. Some people state they feel better when they decrease their intake of protein, carbohydrates, or total calories.

There has been some research using these diets in rheumatoid arthritis. One study tested 10 weeks of diet with no red meat, fruit, dairy products, herbs, spices, preservatives, additives, or alcohol. There was no evidence of a strong difference in arthritis symptoms on that diet although 2 people improved enough to continue the diet. This and other studies have suggested that perhaps some persons do in fact respond to certain changes in the diet, but it is not predictable.

Another more recent study used combinations of wheat, rice, milk, and nonvegetarian food. It found that in many people, arthritis worsened when one or more of these foods was added to the diet. There was a lot of individual variation by elimination of each of the different items in the diet.

We suggest that if your arthritis seems to improve by removing or adding any specific foods, then a trial of a few months might be worthwhile. If it is successful in your case, it can be continued.

New Studies on Omega 3

One of the most exciting areas of diet and arthritis in recent years has been the discovery that some foods can actually reduce inflammation in the body. This was found in Eskimos, who normally have a diet rich in certain fish. Their diet usually contains more protein, less saturated fat, and more polyunsaturated fat. It is interesting to note that rheumatoid arthritis is reported to be less common in Eskimos.

The most common diet in our culture is higher in animal protein. This leads to products in the body which *increase* the inflammatory response. If the diet contains a higher amount of fats found in certain fish (marine lipids) then the body makes products that have *less* inflammatory action.

These (lipids) are called *N-3* or *omega-3 fatty acids*. The most widely known of these in fish oil is EPA (eicosapentaenoic acid) which is available without prescription. The other main omega-3 fatty acid in fish oil is DHA (docosahexaenoic acid). Not all fish contain these specific omega-3 fatty acids.

Some research has already shown that in some rheumatoid arthritis patients who took higher amounts of these fish oil supplements, joint pain and fatigue improved. In other tests, joint swelling and stiffness in the morning improved. As a result, fish oil supplements to the diet in rheumatoid arthritis are recommended by some researchers. No definite dose has yet been established. These supplements are available over the counter. It has been estimated that about 100 grams of herring often gives about the same amount of EPA as many treatments. When used, fish oil is recommended as an addition to the basic treatment program. It should not replace other treatment until the longer term benefits are known. With moderate amounts no serious side effects are known so far.

Proper Nutrition Vital in Treatment

Some practical ideas not to be overlooked in severe arthritis are the need for adequate nutrition intake. The body's nutrition can greatly affect its ability to respond to disease and infection. If weight loss occurs, it may be necessary to increase calorie intake as well as control the disease. Calories should be increased until the proper weight is gained.

If chewing is difficult because of painful jaws or neck, liquid protein supplements and soft foods are needed. If hands are severely affected, then finger foods that are easy to handle without falling apart are excellent.

In cases of poor appetite, try to emphasize "nutrient-dense foods." These foods are loaded with vitamins and minerals, and have fewer "empty" calories. For example, a snack of 12 ounces of carbonated drink has little nutrition but about the same calories as an open-faced grilled cheese sandwich with lowfat cheese. The cheese sandwich is more nutrient dense. Liquid protein supplements are another easy way to provide excellent nutrition in a small volume each day. These are available at drugstores and grocery stores.

Some people have allergies to certain foods. The exact role of food allergies in arthritis is not known. Some people are sensitive to dairy products, nitrates, black walnuts, alfalfa, and other foods. However, at this time, it is thought that food allergies are not a major part of the cause or treatment in most people with arthritis.

Various vitamins and minerals have been suggested as treatment in arthritis, especially more severe rheumatoid arthritis. Vitamin C, zinc, vitamin B, and other vitamins have been used in the past, but no hard evidence for their usefulness is available.

Folk Medicine Diets

There are many folk medicine diets that have not been tested in the same ways the omega-3 fatty acids have been. One folk medicine diet includes elimination of white flour and all sweets (except honey). It recommends eating meat once a week and fish often. There are other diet recommendations. Diets such as these are usually quite healthy and are certainly not harmful.

Nonstandard Treatment

Nonstandard treatments for arthritis have been used for centuries. These treatments are often passed along through the generations by word of mouth, and most of these treatments have some things in common.

- The treatments usually offer quick relief or cure.
- They usually are easy to do.
- They almost always have not been tested in standard ways required by governments for new treatments.
- They are often promoted as good treatments which the medical community is trying to "cover up."
- In many cases, there is a "vendor" nearby willing to sell the treatment.

Some people try these treatments out of frustration over the constant pain. After all, it is hard to turn down what seems like a quick and easy solution. And the person who offers the treatment may expect the person with arthritis to try it and be grateful.

We do not discourage these nonstandard treatments if they are harmless and will not delay proper treatment of the arthritis. In fact, often these nonstandard ways of treating arthritis may give some people peace of mind to know they have not missed an easy answer to their pain. Also, it may give a person more peace from the family member or friend who offers the treatment!

Some nonstandard treatments are definitely not harmful, not expensive, and can easily be added to a basic treatment program for arthritis. You might consider that some treatments are like chicken soup—they won't hurt, and they might help. Just remember to keep up the basic treatment program if you do choose to add a nonstandard treatment.

Arthritis sufferers must become experts so they can manage their treatment properly. It is important to consider the following before using any nonstandard treatment that is not recommended by your physician:

- Ask questions about the treatment including how old it is, what tests have been done, and what the side effects might be.

- Find out what the chances of improvement might be, just as in any other treatment for arthritis.

- There are over 100 kinds of arthritis—does the treatment claim to help *every* kind?

- If the treatment does not help all types of arthritis, does it help *your* kind of arthritis?

Once you have the available facts, you can protect yourself from useless treatments, especially if they distract you from the task of controlling your arthritis.

Let's look at a few of the nonstandard treatments for arthritis.

Antibiotics

Antibiotics have been tried in arthritis, especially rheumatoid arthritis, in the hope that if an infection is the cause, it might be eliminated. Rheumatoid arthritis sometimes begins with fever and other problems that suggest infection of some kind. Also, in people who already have rheumatoid arthritis, an infection may seem to cause a flare up of the arthritis. Researchers have not been able to prove that an infection actually causes rheumatoid arthritis.

Tetracycline has recently been suggested to be a good treatment for rheumatoid arthritis. The claim was made without adequate testing in patients. As is common, the claim was very definite and left little doubt that the results would be excellent.

This treatment is harmless enough that a trial may give a person peace of mind. If there is not a danger (such as allergy) from the tetracycline, then we try to set a time when the treatment will be judged (the claim is that it takes 6 months). If there is no improvement, the treatment is stopped. The basic treatment program should be continued.

Other antibiotics which have been said to work in rheumatoid arthritis are metronidazole and clotrimazole. These claims have been made over the past 15 years or so but have gradually faded away.

Remember that antibiotics are necessary treatment in some kinds of arthritis. Certain infections can cause arthritis. These are very specific types of arthritis and need proper diagnosis. For example, Lyme Arthritis is best treated with antibiotics.

DMSO (Dimethyl Sulfoxide)

DMSO has been used for years in the treatment of muscle strain and sprains in horses. It is used in humans for treatment of some bladder diseases. It has been used with some benefit in the treatment of injuries to muscles and tendons, especially athletic injuries. In injuries, it is applied to the painful area. It is *not* taken internally.

A few years ago DMSO became a popular treatment for arthritis. It was said to be effective in many kinds of arthritis, especially rheumatoid arthritis. Because of this publicity, DMSO has been used by many people with arthritis and related problems. An impure form of DMSO is sold in hardware and other stores that some have used instead of the more pure form. When applied to the skin, DMSO penetrates and is absorbed into the blood. It causes a breath odor somewhat like garlic that is very distinctive. The skin may become irritated where it is used.

DMSO has been injected into veins, which is much more dangerous because it may cause liver or other internal organ damage. DMSO injected into the veins is an example of a non-standard treatment that should be avoided because it may be harmful.

It was difficult to find research to prove or disprove whether DMSO was effective so the U.S. Food and Drug Administration asked a group of scientists to look at all the reports. They found "suggestive" evidence that DMSO might be helpful in some problems, such as acute injuries, painful shoulders (for example, bursitis), and possibly in pain relief in rheumatoid arthritis. They suggested that considering the possible benefits and side effects, it should not be formally approved for use in arthritis until more research was done to prove its effectiveness and define its limitations.

Despite its temporary popularity a few years ago, DMSO is now not very widely used. Those who felt some benefit at first have used it less and less, apparently because of waning effect. The wave of popularity was followed by little use as the limited long-term value for arthritis patients became apparent.

Acupuncture

In acupuncture, very fine needles are inserted into certain areas of the body to produce an effect—in arthritis, relief of pain and swelling. Some research has shown improvement in pain control in rheumatoid arthritis patients even though there was no great effect on swelling. In osteoarthritis and shoulder bursitis, there has been less clear benefit. Overall, there is no definite evidence that acupuncture is an important part of the treatment of arthritis.

Until there is specific evidence to prove whether acupuncture is of benefit, we suggest the following approach. If properly done by a qualified person, acupuncture can be safe. If there is reasonable benefit in an individual patient, it can be used. The basic treatment program should be continued.

Creams, Lotions, and Liniments

Creams, lotions, and liniments are widely advertised for use in arthritis, painful shoulder bursitis, and other conditions. It is hard to show in research that there is a clear advantage to these treatments. But since they are not harmful when used as directed by their makers, there is no objection to their use. Most people try one or more of these creams, lotions, or oils. They can be continued if there is improvement in comfort or if exercise and activity become easier. Many common types of creams, lotions, and rubs are available at your drugstore.

Extracts, Venoms, and Bites

There have been reports of the benefit of snake venom, bee venom, and bee bites for arthritis, especially rheumatoid arthritis. Most of the evidence is in folk medicine although bee venom has been used in some areas of the Far East, Europe, and South America.

In the past few years, researchers have found new evidence that may show that bee venom has an anti-inflammatory effect in arthritis. It was shown to improve arthritis in rats.

Other researchers have found that treatment with extracts from a certain ant improved pain and swelling in people with arthritis. The ant extract was shown to have some specific anti-inflammatory actions.

It is likely that there will be more information in the future about bees, bee venom, ants, and arthritis. It is possible that some forms of these treatments may help people with arthritis.

Herbal Remedies

Herbal remedies have been used for generations in the treatment of arthritis. They may be used in teas, soups, or taken directly. A common ingredient in many is alfalfa.

Some herbal remedies are more popular in certain areas and cultures. Most are not harmful, but no definite positive effect on arthritis has been shown.

Hormone Therapy

The use of hormone therapy in women and men with arthritis received publicity about 15 years ago. It was claimed that the female hormones estrogen and progesterone in women (and male hormone testosterone and progesterone in men) improved or cured osteoarthritis and rheumatoid arthritis. This was not proven in any scientific way and has received little attention since then.

Vinegar and Honey

One folk medicine belief is that people with arthritis don't produce enough acid in their stomachs. Apple cider vinegar is used to provide the acid. The vinegar is said to make the tissues less tender, more elastic, improve the disposition, help constipation, improve the health of the skin, prevent growth of harmful germs, change the blood flow to the digestive organs and other actions. Vinegar and water is used to soak the hands and feet.

Honey is also used in the treatment of arthritis and other problems in some folk medicine. Honey is said to improve digestion. It is said to relieve pain in arthritis, attract fluid, help the body destroy harmful germs, provide nutrients, have a laxative effect, and have the effect of a sedative. The apple cider vinegar and honey is mixed in water and taken at meals or other times.

Iodine and kelp tablets are also a part of the treatment of arthritis according to some folk medicine.

When used in moderate amounts, there is no evidence that these treatments are harmful. Some people feel more peace of mind after they have tried this sort of treatment, just in case it helps their arthritis pain.

Green-Lipped Mussel Extract

An extract of the green-lipped mussel was promoted as a treatment for arthritis a few years ago. No specific differences in the types of arthritis it treated were noted. It was said to be an effective medicine that was being suppressed by organized medicine. The proof that it worked was that it had been given to persons with arthritis who reported that they felt better. And many of the persons who gave the proof were selling the remedy. Little was heard about the mussel extract after a few months.

Copper Bracelets

Copper bracelets are commonly used by arthritis sufferers. It is their hope that the copper is in some way absorbed and has a beneficial effect on arthritis. One survey found up to 45 percent of patients had used a copper bracelet at one time, while another survey found they were rarely used. These bracelets are not harmful and if a person feels they give benefit, it is hard to discourage their use if other proper treatment is continued.

Spas, Baths, and Mud Packs

The use of spas and baths is one of the oldest treatments for arthritis sufferers (this is called balneotherapy). The Romans built baths to provide warm pools to treat arthritis. The moist heat provided relief even if only temporary, just as the moist heat used in today's treatments. Many spas are still active and in many ways function as a form of physical therapy by giving moist heat and exercise to their users.

A recent study used sulphur bath and mud packs given for 2 weeks at a spa hotel. Some improvement in pain, stiffness, and patient ease in performing daily activities was found using daily hot sulphur baths, daily mud packs, or both. No severe side effects were found. Some arthritis experts feel that this type of treatment should not be used during more active or severe rheumatoid arthritis.

Prayer

Some nonstandard treatments are even older. Prayer was used by over 40 percent of people with arthritis in one recent survey. There have been some attempts to compare treatment using prayer to treatment without prayer. As might be expected, it was difficult to make any firm scientific conclusions. In the survey noted above, over *half* of the people rated prayer as very helpful.

Relaxation and Meditation

Some people claim that relaxation and meditation help with the pain associated with arthritis. These alone times could be spent watching the sunset in the evening, listening to a favorite tape collection, or even taking a short walk in the evenings. The meditation is used to relax those muscles that are held so tight during stressful, painful moments.

Others—Not Recommended

Every arthritis sufferer has heard of other remedies promoted to give relief. Some of those reported over the past few years and definitely not recommended include rubbing joints with kerosene, oil, or brake fluid. Cocaine, vaccines, the extract of yucca plants, and other remedies have been claimed over the years, but have not been proven to be at all helpful. There are also claims that tooth fillings for dental cavities may cause arthritis and other diseases and should be replaced.

The Goal Is to Protect Yourself

Some treatments that are harmless can be used if there is benefit. When these are used, try to set a time to expect some improvement in arthritis pain or stiffness or some other detectable way. If there is no improvement, the treatment can be stopped.

Treatments that are nonstandard and unproven, and that

might be harmful should be avoided. There are times when it is difficult to tell whether a new treatment is another unproven remedy that will disappear or whether it is the new break-through you have been waiting for. Press reports may unin-tentionally make the treatment appear more positive and useful than it will turn out to be over a longer period of time. Some examples of these were mentioned above. How can a person who suffers from arthritis tell which treatments to take advan-tage of early?

The Arthritis Foundation (See page 201) is the best source for information about new or unproven treatments. Local chap-ters or the national office can provide up-to-date, honest and thorough information to allow you to decide about new treat-ments. Also, talk with your physician for advice on the risks and benefits of a new treatment. Then you will be able to benefit as early as possible from new developments in arthritis. But you will also be able to protect yourself from unwanted effects of unproven remedies.

CHAPTER EIGHT

Managing Stress and Chronic Pain

Coping effectively with stress is an important part of any disease and arthritis is no exception. High levels of stress cause "wear and tear" on the body and contribute to the development of certain illnesses over time. Excessive stress can aggravate existing medical problems and cause an increase in symptoms and difficulties. With arthritis, stress can lead to more frequent and intense pain and make it harder to handle other problems brought on by the illness.

Stress is the word used to describe the many demands and pressures that all people experience to one degree or another. These demands require us to change or adapt in some fashion and may be physical or emotional in nature. For example, being stuck in slow-moving traffic requires that we change our expectations about arriving at our destination at a certain time. Similarly, the stress of going through a critical job interview requires that we maintain a relaxed, yet self-assured and confident approach in order to do our best and make a favorable impression.

People with arthritis are faced with special demands and pressures from a chronic illness that may require from only a few up to major changes in lifestyle or daily habits. Pain is among the most common symptoms experienced by arthritis patients. The task of coping with daily pain often given rise to stress that can actually make the pain more frequent and intense. When you are in pain, the body has a natural tendency to tighten up—Muscles can become tense and rigid, causing additional strain and pressure on already tender joints or areas of inflammation. This muscle tension causes the pain to be worse, which leads to additional stress and tension, and even more discomfort.

Chronic pain of arthritis, along with other special problems such as loss of independence, work adjustment difficulties, and preoccupation or worry about the future can combine to cause depression and other emotional reactions which further limit your ability to deal effectively with daily living. Depression is not a weakness; rather it is a common response to chronic stress in which people come to feel helpless and hopeless for relief.

Stress can show itself through a wide variety of physical changes and emotional responses. Stress symptoms vary greatly from one person to the next. Perhaps the most universal sign of stress is a feeling of being pressured or overwhelmed. Some other signs and symptoms of stress are:

- Chronic fatigue
- Loss of interest or enjoyment
- Concentration difficulties
- Muscle tension
- Impatience
- Irritability or easy to anger
- Difficulty sleeping
- Change in appetite
- Nervousness, edginess
- Withdrawal
- Trembling, sweaty hands

If you recognize many or most of these characteristics in yourself, chances are good that your level of stress is excessive. Learning to identify the ways in which your body and mind show stress is the first step in "managing the self" and reducing external demands and pressures, as well as those that we place on ourselves.

The Stress of Chronic Pain

The person with arthritis typically deals with pain on a daily basis and the reason for the pain is genuine—there is something wrong in the body. The last thing you want to hear is, "I think it might be a good idea for you to speak with someone about your stress." You immediately recognize that "someone" is either a psychiatrist, psychologist, or a counselor of some type—more commonly known as a "shrink." You may be offended by the implication that the pain is "in your head," and you may even become suspicious that this person does not believe that you are really feeling the degree of pain you describe.

If this has already happened to you or if it happens in the future, take a minute to explore your thoughts so that you can approach this subject in a rational manner. Let's examine some of the thoughts that may occur.

- *He thinks I'm making up my pain.*

  It is highly unlikely that your physician, friend, or whoever has recommended that you receive help believes you are *not* in pain. If you immediately become defensive and imagine the worst, this throws up roadblocks to any help you could receive by considering the impact of your emotional state on your pain. There is pain associated with arthritis—that is a given fact that few would dispute. Do not allow yourself to avoid the possibility of lessening the pain by assuming that others disbelieve or under rate your pain.

- *He doesn't understand what it is like to be in pain like this.*

  It is true that those who are suggesting that you see a counselor may not have experienced the day-to-day debilitating pain that you constantly endure. However, lack of personal experience does not mean that their suggestions are not valid. Experienced professionals have formed a base of knowledge over the years, and they have seen the positive results of gaining control over emotions. They do not have to feel exactly as you do to make a valid recommendation for your welfare.

- *He thinks I could do more if I would only try.*

  You know you have tried, and you are likely to be turned off by the implication that you have not put forth the effort. But did you listen carefully? Did the person say you have not tried? Probably not. More often than not this is an interpretation that you have placed on the situation. You *are* trying, but you may not have tried or worked at your emotions from the standpoint that you can be in control. You have the ability to change your thought, and thus change your perception of the pain.

The Role of Psychology in Chronic Arthritis Pain

All comprehensive inpatient and outpatient chronic pain programs include a psychological and/or behavioral component. This is because it is widely accepted that your emotional status has a significant effect on both your perception of the pain and your ability to develop appropriate coping strategies.

All people with pain are stressed. This stress makes it more difficult to handle everyday issues, much less crisis situations that may arise. Thus, the role of psychological counseling in a pain management program is to help the individual develop appropriate and functional coping strategies to deal with all of these issues. Psychological intervention is an accepted component for everyone—*not* just the ones who have "psychological problems."

The inclusion of psychological intervention consists of methods/techniques that people with arthritis can use either within or outside of a formalized program. In most cases, it is important that the therapist performing these services be trained in the area of pain management. Some of these options include the following:

- *Individual Counseling*

  This is a one-on-one session with a therapist in which individual problem areas are addressed. This may include specific help with alleviating depression, anxiety, or stress, along with a multitude of other problem areas addressed more specifically in the following section.

- *Family Counseling*

   Your pain with arthritis can affect the entire family. It is often necessary for family members to be involved in understanding your limitations and the impact this may have on your family's lifestyle. Family members can have the best of intentions, but without specific guidance, they may unknowingly make things worse. Family meetings are a way of helping everyone deal with the stress of your disability.

- *Group Counseling*

   There is no one who can better understand you than another arthritic patient. Group sessions allow for the sharing of feelings, as well as the development of effective coping strategies. As you become emotionally healthy regarding your condition, this allows you the opportunity to share your success and optimism with others. The give and take of group meetings is often the most productive way to revamp your thought processes.

Biofeedback

Relaxation is an accepted form of managing stress. Many chronic pain programs teach patients to relax in order to reduce their pain levels. This can be accomplished through the use of progressive relaxation, guided imagery, or the use of a medical technique called *biofeedback.* You are connected to a machine that informs you and your therapist when you are physically relaxing your body. This can be accomplished by either reading the tension in your muscles, the amount of sweat produced, or the measurement of finger temperature. Any one or all of these readings can indicate to a trained biofeedback therapist if you are learning to relax. The skill of relaxing can then be used outside of the therapist's office when you encounter the day-to-day stresses of life. Some therapists recommend relaxation tapes that can be listened to at home to practice relaxation techniques.

Emotional and/or Behavioral Areas to Address in Pain Management

Working with people with arthritis, it becomes quite evident that you share a large number of problems in your life with others. The types of arthritis are varied, the structures of families are different, and the tolerance you possess for pain runs from low to high endurance. In spite of all these variations, the problems you experience are often similar to other patients in effect on you and your loved ones.

It is not fun to be in pain, and at times you may have felt or even expressed the fact that "a life with pain is *no* life at all." Your problems are *real* and are often devastating to your outlook on life and your daily activities. Going through some of these negative areas, you can learn effective coping techniques that lead to a positive *winning* attitude.

Read each topic with an open mind and explore ways in which *you* can have an impact in your life. This is an area where *you* can change. These *are* alternatives to relying solely on the medical interventions discussed in other chapters in this book, especially when many of the other avenues have been exhausted. Not all of these problem areas may apply to your type or stage of arthritis. We do, however, recommend that you read and think carefully about each emotion discussed. It may be something that you will have to face in the future or it may help you help others.

Anger/Irritability

Most people feel some degree of anger at the fact that they have arthritis. Some have used the anger in a positive manner, some have ignored the anger, and some have let these angry feelings consume their whole being. You can understand these feelings better and replace the energy you spend being angry with positive actions to make your life pleasurable.

Upfront anger is expressed directly toward the person or situation at which you are angry. This type of anger, if not belabored, is most acceptable. *Displaced anger* originates from strong feelings toward a person or event, but is directed toward another person or event. For example, your physician may have suggested that you see a counselor to help you learn to relax. This suggestion that the pain might "be in your head" makes you furious. Instead of screaming at the doctor and telling him that he's an idiot, you scream at your spouse, expressing displaced anger. *Inward anger* is unexpressed, either verbally or nonverbally. Instead of speaking about your anger, you let it boil up inside and eat away at your whole being.

You have a right to be angry, but you do *not* have a right to devastate yourself and others while expressing this anger. By holding onto angry feelings, you prevent yourself from moving forward to a more positive outlook.

Coping Strategies for Anger/Irritability

1. Accept the fact that anger is a human emotion that you are entitled to feel at times.
2. If anger is consuming your entire day, come to grips with the fact that you need to explore some avenues for behavioral change.
3. Remember that constantly being in an angry state is detrimental to your overall health.
4. When your anger gets out of control, apologize to those you may have hurt.
5. Whenever possible, do *not* let yourself get into situations that you know will be unpleasant.
6. Ask your physician for a recommendation of a professional who can assist you in relaxing and reducing the tension that occurs from anger.

Loss of Independence

The pain associated with arthritis often leads to a loss of independence in your life. The degree of this loss varies with the frequency of pain, intensity of pain, and your personality structure. We all have different tolerance levels and methods of handling our problems.

If you are the type who has always relied on other people, the entrance of chronic pain into your life has probably *increased* your level of dependence. You may have found this very comfort-able; however, chances are your family is feeling overwhelmed by your needs.

On the other hand, you may be the type of person who has prided herself on never having to rely on others. If so, having to give up some of this self-sufficiency has probably wreaked havoc with your self-concept. You may even find yourself going with-out some necessities just because you will *not* ask someone else to help.

Coping Strategies for Loss of Independence

1. Do not confuse what you *cannot* do with what you *can* do but are trying to avoid because of pain.
2. If you have the financial means, purchase the services you need instead of relying on family members. The family may be very willing, but over time this dependency can lead to feelings of resentment.
3. Try to do something new each week that you previously asked others to do for you.
4. *Never* let your family think you equate their love with the amount of help they give.
5. If you are doing everything you are physically capable of doing, do *not* feel guilty asking for assistance with the things you absolutely cannot do.
6. Remember that the more you can do for yourself, the better you will feel about yourself.
7. Never use guilt to make your family feel bad that they are not doing enough to help you.

Loss of Control

Loss of control over your life can include a loss of much more than independence. You now find that your activities no longer depend upon your intelligence, financial ability, perse-verance, or desire. You are now limited by what your pain will allow you to do. It is a feeling that cannot be easily understood by those who have not experienced the debilitating effects of arthritis. There is a fine line between what you think you can-not control and what you absolutely cannot control. The key to dealing effectively with this problem is to make sure you understand where these two areas differ.

Coping Strategies for Loss of Control

1. Determine what things you can control and make positive steps toward that goal, rather than dwelling upon your lack of control in other areas.

2. Make a list of things you want to change, then divide them into two categories: (a) those things I can control, and (b) those things I cannot control. With the help of therapists, family, or friends, begin to work on those aspects that can be controlled.

3. If you find yourself becoming extremely agitated and/or stressed over a situation that is out of your control, try to refocus your thoughts. If this does not work, ask for help from a professional.

4. Never consider yourself weak if you think you need help with accepting some loss of control. The weak individuals are really those who refuse to ask for help. Asking for help is, in fact, helping yourself.

5. Start working each week on a new action that will help you gain control. If you have trouble deciding what these should be, ask a counselor or trusted friend to help you prioritize your list of actions that are possibly within your control.

6. Throw your pessimistic attitude away. You *can* gain better control, but you must work for it.

Acceptance

The ultimate goal for you as a chronic pain patient is to reach the point where you can accept the arthritis and are ready to make modifications to handle it within your life. The flip side of this acceptance is denial. Denial is the behavior that works at complete odds with any type of rehabilitation effort. If you are not willing to admit that nonmedical issues are affecting your pain, then you will have no reason to engage in any type of rehabilitative therapy.

Denial or nonacceptance is often a way to preserve our self-esteem. We may think that, if we admit that anything other than a physical problem is increasing our pain, everyone will say that *all* our pain is "psychological" or "in our head." This is not the case. It is known that stress factors at home and on the job can have definite effects on many things—including pain.

Coping Strategies for Reaching Acceptance

1. Keep a daily log of your actions, feelings, and intensity of pain. Ask a counselor or someone trained in pain management to analyze the log.
2. Work on accepting the level of pain that you are experiencing and focus your efforts on managing your life with the existing pain. Any decrease in pain can then be an unexpected surprise rather than an expected occurrence.
3. Do *not* equate psychological assistance with the assumption that people think your pain is in your head.
4. Accept the possibility that you could benefit by stress management techniques.
5. Keep an open mind to nonmedical alternatives such as biofeedback, relaxation, and counseling.

Depression

If you have not experienced some degree of depression with the pain associated with arthritis, then your situation is unusual. It is common for individuals in pain to encounter some degree of depression. The intensity and frequency can vary from momentary sadness to complete immobilization and suicidal thoughts.

You may be the type of person who considers himself very strong and not *subject* to emotional reactions such as depression. Just because you think you are not depressed, however, does not mean you are not experiencing depression. Depressive symptoms can include mood swings, loss of interest in activities such as hobbies and going out of the house, avoidance of special friends, excessive sleep or lack thereof, reduced or increased appetite and difficulty concentrating.

On the other hand, you may be well aware that you are depressed due to uncontrollable tearfulness, feelings of helplessness and/or hopelessness, loss of self-worth, and suicidal thoughts or plans. If this is the case, you must contact a professional—do not fight getting help.

Coping Strategies for Combatting Depression

1. Never keep suicidal thoughts to yourself. Let someone help you.
2. See a qualified mental health specialist if depression is immobilizing you.
3. Never use alcohol or non-prescribed drugs to combat depression.
4. Seek counseling to explore the relationship between depression and pain. It can be very confusing to you and others.
5. Exercise is a great cure for depression. Determine what you can do medically to become active.
6. Never stay in bed all day unless advised by your physician.

Anxiety and Fears

Arthritic patients have legitimate fears of the future—How much worse will I get? Will I be able to keep my job? Can I continue to care for my children? Will I be an invalid?

If one were to become obsessed with these issues it would be very difficult to move in a positive direction. Instead, you need to *acknowledge your fears* and *channel your energy* into positive action to either stop the deteriorating process or to slow the rate of change. Spending time worrying about facts that cannot be changed only wastes precious time that can be spent on positive actions.

Coping Strategies for Alleviating Anxiety and Fears

1. Identify anxiety provoking situations and try to avoid them if possible.
2. Discuss your concerns with a professional—*do not* expect a family member to be your therapist.
3. Have an open mind about interventions that can help you relax, such as biofeedback.
4. Join a support group of arthritic patients.
5. Ask your physician to explain to your family why there are some days you do better than others.

Loss of Self-Esteem

The pain of arthritis can lead to loss of job, decreased contact with friends, and reduction in leisure activities. For many of us, our entire self-esteem is wrapped up in one or all of these aspects. Now, when someone says "What do you do?" you may not respond with "I'm a clerk" or "I'm a manager." Instead, you think to yourself "I'm a failure" or "I sit home all day." When you no longer have an occupation with which to identify, your self-worth may suffer.

For you, being with friends and doing things for them and your family may have been your identity. Instead of being able to take an entire meal over to a sick friend or driving your neighbor to have his car fixed, *you* are the one who needs help. If you have been a very independent person, this switch to dependency has probably taken its toll on your self-confidence.

Coping Strategies for Combatting Low Self-Esteem

1. Make a list of all your good qualities.
2. Take your focus off the negative aspect of your life.
3. Remember that your family did not love you only for the paycheck you brought home.
4. Allow yourself to consider less demanding jobs that would occupy your time and make you feel worthwhile.
5. Do *not* avoid social interactions. In the end, this only makes things worse.
6. Try to do as many things for yourself as you can. You will feel better the more independent you become.

Guilt

Unless you are the type of person who enjoys having time off from work and being dependent on others, you are going to have some degree of guilt regarding the circumstances of your life. Guilt generally centers around three major areas: (1) Money, (2) pulling your own weight, or (3) infringing upon other people's time for help.

If you were the major breadwinner and have not been working for an extended period of time, you may be feeling guilty about not providing for your family as you think you should. This type of guilt can also be felt by secondary breadwinners, or even just because extensive medical bills have added an additional financial burden.

You may have found those jobs within the home for which you were entirely responsible are now impossible to complete. This leaves you with a sense of shirking your responsibilities. Furthermore, it may frustrate you that no one else does them, and you may find yourself getting angry at others for unfinished jobs. When you realize that those duties were always yours, guilt may set in.

Finally, not only can you not perform your usual duties, but sometimes family members have to take time to help you with simple things that you could always do for yourself before. If you dislike that dependent feeling, you are bound to become riddled with guilt.

Coping Strategies for Dealing with Guilt

1. Accept guilt as a normal human feeling over which you have minimal control.
2. Try your best to do as many things for yourself as you can.
3. Never ask someone else to do something you can do.
4. Do not live in the past—work on changing the future.

Stress

You may not have known the true meaning of *stress* until you lived with chronic pain for a period of time. "Stressed Out" describes the impact that life stressors have on you, including anxiety, tension, high blood pressure, depression, anger, distractibility, disorientation, and an entire host of physical problems including an increase in pain. You, as an arthritis patient, experience stressors across all aspects of your life. There are physical stressors (the pain), social stressors (loss of friends and activities), work stressors (loss of job or difficulty working), and family stressors (feeling of dependency on others).

You have every right to be stressed, but you can do something about it. Two basic methods for coping with stress are relaxation and the use of social support—trusted friends. Relaxation involves more than getting away from stressful situations;

it is more a mental approach to doing things rather than any specific activity or thing you do. Relaxation is a positive and satisfy-
ing feeling in which you experience a sense of inner calm and
peace of mind.

Relaxation is a skill that is learned through practice and
rehearsal. The key to getting the best results from attempts at
relaxation is to find those activities that give you pleasure. When
you pursue them, direct your energies toward total mental and
physical well-being.

Here are some possibilities to consider:

- Try some mental exercise to create a sense of peace and
  tranquility in body and mind. One exercise involves concentration on relaxing successive sets of muscles from the tips
  of your toes to the muscles in the face and neck. Other
  techniques include getting fully involved with a good book,
  drifting off into a quiet state with music, or imagining a
  beautiful scene or drawing and losing yourself in it.

- Creative activities such as painting, pottery, knitting, and
  cooking for fun can give a sense of accomplishment along
  with the peaceful relaxation of concentration on something
  you wish to do.

After discovering your favorite relaxation activity, plan to
devote at least 30 minutes per day to pursuing it. Don't rush
it—learning relaxation skills requires a commitment of both time
and energy to achieve the most benefit—it's worth it!

Sharing your problems and feelings with others is often
helpful in reducing tension and providing an outlet for internal
feelings of pressure. There is comfort in knowing that others
care and will take time to listen—although they may not have
all the answers or simple solutions to problems. Seek out a
person in whom you have confidence and trust—whether it is
your spouse, other family member, clergyperson, or next door
neighbor and begin to talk about what troubles you. Support
groups for arthritis patients provide an excellent source of
helpful information and mutual understanding of the special
demands and pressures of living with arthritis. It helps to
know you're not alone with your problem, and the experience

of others may suggest new ideas of approaches to solving nagging problems.

Should you find it difficult to get a handle on your stress and feel increasingly overwhelmed and helpless, talk to your physician and work together on solving the problem. A referral to a psychologist or psychiatrist who specializes in evaluating and treating stress-related difficulties may be helpful in individualizing a stress management program to deal with your symptoms. If you feel that stress is managing you to a greater and greater degree, don't hesitate to seek professional help. Coping more effectively with stress will assist you in reducing pain, feeling better overall, and dealing more positively with your arthritis.

Coping Strategies for Decreasing Stress

1. Enroll in a stress management class or seminar offered at your local community mental health center.
2. If you are experiencing physical symptoms of stress, such as high blood pressure, headaches, or anxiety attacks, be sure to consult your physician.
3. An individual counselor might be helpful in learning to relax and manage your specific stress.
4. Consider special techniques, such as biofeedback, to provide you with tools to lower body tension or raise temperature levels.
5. Stress management books and/or relaxation tapes are available at local book stores.
6. Examine your life carefully. Make a comprehensive list of all the things that stress you out. Eliminate or avoid those that are not absolutely necessary. Try to modify the others.

Fatigue

After having pain for six months or more, you are very likely to be worn to a frazzle, both physically and mentally. There are days when you feel that it would be impossible to move another muscle, even if you had to. You are tired of trips to the doctor, not being able to go out with friends, constantly hurting with every move, and just plain tired of being tired.

As strange as this may sound, the cure for fatigue is exercise. Many people do not believe this because they are so accustomed to solving fatigue with rest. However, it is exercise that builds up your stamina—not rest.

Coping Strategies for Fatigue

1. Consult your physician for an appropriate exercise regime.
2. If your physician agrees, participate in physical therapy with a therapist who is familiar with chronic pain.
3. Utilize relaxation techniques for insomnia. If you are unfamiliar with these, consult a counselor.
4. Stress leads to fatigue—so avoid it or at least learn to manage it.
5. Anger and tension also lead to fatigue. Avoid situations that induce these types of feelings.
6. Exercise regularly as recommended by your physician—no exceptions, please!

There may be other issues facing you. Because of the stresses that may develop due to arthritis, you may experience everyday stresses in an ineffective or exaggerated manner. You can exhibit control, and you can make changes in both your thinking and acting. Do not feel that you must do this alone. There are trained professionals ready to guide you and your family in a positive direction. Do not be afraid or ashamed to ask for help.

CHAPTER NINE

Back Pain: A Common Problem

Back pain is one of the most common health problems. There are many causes, including arthritis, simple strain, osteoporosis and ruptured disc.

Back pain may be mild and might last only a few minutes. Or, the pain can be more severe and may last for months or years. It can make work difficult. In fact, back pain is the most common cause of loss of work after the common cold!

What causes severe back pain? Can these attacks be prevented? What can be done when the back pain lasts for weeks, months, or even years?

It helps to look at two types of lower back pain. The first type is the pain that strikes suddenly or comes on over one or two days. This is ACUTE back pain. It usually lasts from hours up to a few weeks. The second type is CHRONIC back pain which lasts for weeks, months or years. Let's look at these two types of back pain and how you can control them.

Acute Back Pain

Acute back pain can be almost unbearable. It can be sharp, dull, or aching. It is most often felt as a deep pain in the lower part of the back. The pain may be felt more on the right, on the left, or in the center of the lower back. It may come and go, but it is usually constant. Acute back pain usually lasts from a few hours to a few weeks.

This severe, acute pain may come on after an injury, but even more commonly has no noticeable cause. It may be made worse by coughing or sneezing. The pain often prevents sleep at night. It is often improved by lying flat on your back although it may be difficult to find a comfortable position.

The pain may travel down one or both legs (Figure 9.1). It can move down the front, side, or back of either leg. When the pain (and sometimes numbness and tingling) travels down the back of one leg it may be called *sciatica*. This name comes from the sciatic nerve that passes down the back of the leg. One description of the feeling of sciatica is "like hot water running down the back of the leg."

There is usually little to see in a person in acute back pain. Walking or bending over are difficult and may be possible only with great effort. Lying quietly without movement is often the only comfortable position.

Causes of Acute Back Pain

The exact causes of acute back pain are not known in most cases. Although it is usually called *acute lumbar strain,* the cause of the strain may be an injury after lifting or more often is not apparent. Some specific medical problems can cause acute back pain and are important to find as early as possible. These include arthritis, internal organ diseases, infections around the spine, cancer, and fracture of the spine.

When should you see your physician for acute back pain? If the pain is severe or happens for the first time then it is reasonable to ask your physician for advice. If the pain lasts more than a few days, it is a good idea to see your physician. Other warning signs that should alert you to get medical evaluation are:

- When the pain is worse with a cough or sneeze
- When it awakens you from sleep

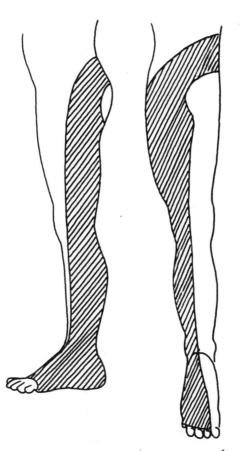

Figure 9.1. Diagram of some areas of leg pain with back pain and sciatica.

- When it becomes difficult to pass urine or have a bowel movement
- When there is loss of control of the urine or bowel movements
- If pain or numbness travels down the leg. (See Figure 9.1.)

These problems may be the earliest signs of serious nerve damage and the need for early treatment.

Tests Used in Diagnosing Acute Back Pain

What tests might be ordered when you have acute back pain? It is surprising, but x-rays of the lower back (lumbar spine) do not usually give much information, although they do help to eliminate other problems such as cancer or fracture of the spine.

Some blood tests or other studies may be ordered if other medical problems are suspected. There are other tests if the pain does not improve with treatment. See page 187.

Treating Acute Back Pain

The good news is that over 80 percent of people with acute back pain improve within about two weeks. The basic treatment program for acute back pain includes brief bed rest, exercises, and medications that may be of several types.

Brief Bed Rest

For many years patients were told to stay in bed for a week or more with acute back pain. It has now been shown that less bed rest may be needed. One study found that 2 days of complete bed rest worked as well as 7 days with reduced activity.

We suggest limited activity or bed rest if needed at first until the pain is controlled enough to allow standing and walking. This usually turns out to be 1 to 3 days. Then a gradual return to walking and usual daily activities can begin. At first, work must be limited to avoid lifting, bending, or prolonged standing or walking. In many cases, work can be adjusted to allow little or no loss of time at work.

Moist Heat and Exercises

As soon as possible, within the first day or two of pain, moist heat and exercises are begun. This usually requires instruction or supervision by a physical therapist so that the pain is not made worse by exercise. Moist heat such as warm towels, warm shower, warm bathtub, hot packs, or moist heating pad may be used. The moist heat is applied to the back for 15 to 20 minutes 2 or 3 times daily.

In some cases of acute back pain, an ice pack (ice in plastic bags or ice bag) may do as well or better than moist heat. Some find it best to alternate ice and heat. Choose what works best for you.

Try doing the exercises while the moist heat or ice is used. This may make it easier, especially when just beginning the exercise program.

Begin with 1 of the first back exercise and gradually increase to one of each exercise (see page 120). Then gradually increase to 2 of each exercise. As there is improvement in pain and the back becomes more flexible and limber, the number of repetitions may be gradually increased. The eventual goal is to be able to comfortably do about 20 repetitions of each exercise twice daily.

There may be a little more discomfort at first when exercises are used early in the course and gradually increased. But some researchers have found the pain relief is often better over a longer period of time when the exercises are started early. It seems that as the back muscles become stronger and more flexible with more endurance, the back pain improves and has less chance of returning.

Medications

Medications of several different types are used in acute back pain. The non-cortisone anti-inflammatory drugs (NSAIDS) are used to decrease the inflammation that is often found in the lower back tissues. These give the best relief when they are used within the first day or two.

Many of this group of medications have been used with success. The advantage of these drugs is the good possibility of relief without sedation or drowsiness. The possible side effects are listed in Table 4.4. Since these medications are often needed for only a few days, the side effects are less common than with long-term use in arthritis. If nausea, heartburn, or indigestion occur, the drug should be stopped.

Muscle relaxants are used when there is muscle spasm in the lower back. In these cases, there may be a lot of discomfort from the muscles that become tightened. Muscle relaxants can give temporary relief of the painful muscle spasms. The most common side effects of these medications are drowsiness and sedation (see page 57).

Pain (analgesic) medications may be needed in acute back pain. These include aspirin, acetaminophen, and stronger pain medications such as the narcotics codeine, propxyphene (Darvon), and derivatives of these drugs. These may help in early severe pain but should be minimized as soon as possible to avoid becoming dependent (see page 56).

Other Types of Treatment

Traction is an older form of treatment that attempts to lower the pressure on the lower back tissues. This requires bed rest and has not been used as often in recent years. Its effectiveness is somewhat controversial and many patients feel it is more trouble than the benefit received.

Back braces and corsets may be tried in acute back pain, but most patients find they are so uncomfortable that they leave them off. A problem with braces and corsets is that to be effective they may be heavy and can be quite uncomfortable. We suggest that if they help the pain, these supports may be used. However, they should be removed for exercises twice daily and should be used only until there is improvement.

Massage may be helpful in acute back pain. This may be performed by a physical therapist or other qualified person such as a massage therapist and may give relief. Manipulation as performed by chiropractors and osteopathic physicians may give short-term relief of pain just as many other forms of treatment. If this treatment gives relief, it should be continued. If there is no improvement, then it may be eliminated just as any other form of treatment that does not prove effective.

Prevention

Once the pain is gone, is there any way to prevent these painful attacks of acute back pain? It turns out that you *can* actually affect what happens in the future. The best plan is to maintain a regular exercise program and to learn what activities increase the risk of a return of the back pain.

When the pain is much better or completely gone, *don't stop the exercise program.* Remember that it takes weeks and months to build stronger muscles. The goal is to make the muscles of the back stronger and more flexible to help prevent future injury and strain. It is not always easy to continue the back exercises when the pain is gone. Try to remember how painful it was—and that a regular back exercise program can help decrease the chance of the pain returning.

Try to stay fit and trim. This means *stay near your ideal body weight.* Excess body weight puts more load and stress on the lower back.

Try to include cardiovascular exercise in your program. This could include beginning a regular walking program, starting with a very short distance each day. Then, gradually increase the distance as long as there is no discomfort. You will be surprised how quickly you can increase the length of the walk. Most important is to do it at least 5 days each week. Other exercise could include swimming, bicycle, or exercise bicycle. An exercise bicycle is easy since it can be done at any time of day or night, regardless of the weather.

Many jobs and daily activities require awkward body positions or stressful lifting positions. Not all of these can be eliminated. You must be in good physical condition to meet these demands. Many of us blame "the job" when we in fact have done little to keep our bodies maintained to perform the task properly.

Many injuries happen to the back when lifting an object. It is important to *lift correctly,* that is:

1. Always try to lift with the legs and not the back. When you lift an object from the floor, you should be close to the object with knees bent and the back relatively straight (in a squat position). The object should be close to your body and not held at arm's length. Raise up using the leg muscles.
2. Never twist when lifting. If you must turn, pivot with the feet.
3. Do not lift objects higher than chest level. If you must reach above your head use a stool.
4. Always be sure of your footing.
5. If an object is too heavy, have someone else help you lift or use a mechanical aid or lever.

Incorrect posture can cause excess strain on the lower back. It is important to know how to *maintain a correct posture.*

1. If your job involves sitting at a desk for long periods of time, stand up for a few minutes every hour or two to stretch backwards or walk.

2. The chair you use at the desk should support the lower back. The feet should comfortably reach the floor.

3. The arms of the chair at the desk should be able to go under the desk to help prevent the position of sitting and leaning forward. In this case, excess stress is put on the lower back. The pressure on the discs in the lower spine has actually been measured to be highest when sitting and leaning forward, less when sitting straight and less when standing. Sitting unsupported may cause up to 40 percent higher pressure on the lumbar disc compared to standing.

4. Use of lumbar supports or cushions can help to maintain the lower back in a natural position and avoid slumping.

If your job or daily activity involves much standing, here are several suggestions:

1. Wear comfortable shoes, usually with low heels. Certainly try to avoid high heel shoes if possible.

2. Stand with one foot "propped" on a box or stool.

3. Hold the abdominal muscles in—avoid the "swayback" position if possible.

4. Try not to stand in only one position for long periods at a time.

5. Try placing a rubber mat in the area you stand to help provide a "cushion" for your feet and back.

For Prevention of Back Pain

1. *Continue* a regular back exercise program.

2. Stay in good physical condition and control your body weight. Include cardiovascular exercise in your program.

3. Lift correctly.

4. Use mechanical lifts and aids if needed.

5. Try to maintain correct posture. Avoid awkward body positions when possible.

6. Let the work site work for you. Pay attention to desk height

and chairs. Organize your work space for the best efficiency and to improve body mechanics.

If the Pain Lasts

After a few weeks, the large majority of persons have relief of acute back pain with this basic treatment program. But what happens if the acute back pain does not improve? If the pain is severe and activity is still severely limited, further evaluation is necessary. If pain remains in the lower back and one or both legs as described in sciatica, further tests are needed.

Further Diagnosis and Treatment of Acute Back Pain

When the pain does not improve, other medical problems must be eliminated. This can usually be done by your physician after discussion and examination followed by blood tests and x-rays. If no other medical problems are found, then one or more of the tests discussed below are used to find the specific cause of the back pain. If a definite cause of the pain can be found, treatment will be more effective.

The most common cause of persistent lower back pain with sciatica is rupture (herniation) of one of the discs between the bones of the lumbar spine. (See Figure 9.2.)

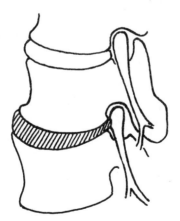

Figure 9.2. Diagram of lumbar disc. The disc material causes pressure on the nearby nerve.

Further Diagnosis and Treatment of Acute Back Pain

Computed Tomographic Scan

Computed tomographic (CT) scan of the lumbar spine can detect the rupture or herniation of a disc in most cases. It also can detect other problems in the spine such as infection, fracture, and cancer. It detects the disc rupture 75 percent or more of the time. Like most tests, it is not perfect. This may occasionally show an abnormal disc when it is actually normal. This test costs approximately $500 to $600 in many areas.

Magnetic Resonance Imaging

Magnetic Resonance Imaging (MRI) is considered by most experts to be as good or better than CT scans for detecting ruptured discs in the lumbar spine. It shows the ruptured disc accurately 90 percent or more of the time.

MRI and CT scan both can be done without admission to the hospital. Both tests can be done without injections of medication or dye and have minimal risk. The cost of MRI is $750 to $900 in most areas.

Myelogram

Myelogram is a test that requires an injection of dye to show the rupture of a disc in the lumbar spine. It detects the rupture in *over* 90 percent of cases. The myelogram has more discomfort and a higher possibility of unwanted side effects. Some experts now recommend MRI of the lumbar spine, then if there is not a clear answer, a myelogram is performed. The cost varies, but is approximately $1200 to $1500. CT scan may be combined with myelogram to improve the accuracy of diagnosis.

Bone Scan

A bone scan is a test that can detect abnormal areas in bones including the spine. This test is used in some cases when there is suspicion of infection, cancer, or fracture. It does not replace the above tests but may add information by eliminating these other serious problems. The cost is approximately $300 to $400.

Other causes of pain in the back with sciatica are less common and are discovered by your physician, often with the help of a consulting specialist. Every person is different and may require a different combination of tests.

Further Treatment of Back Pain Due to Ruptured Discs

Injections

Injections around the spine called epidural injections can be used for relief of pain in persons who have continuous lower back pain. The injection is usually a combination of a local anesthetic and a cortisone derivative. These injections do not cure the ruptured disc but may give pain relief. The effect may not be long-lasting. If the relief is excellent but wears off after a few months or more, the injection is sometimes repeated.

Surgery

The good news is that less than 10 percent of persons with back pain and sciatica need surgery. In those who do not have good relief with the basic treatment program including moist heat, exercises, rest, medications, and injections, surgery may give excellent results.

The main benefits of surgery are pain relief and the return to usual activity more quickly. The results of surgery are good 90 percent of the time when a ruptured disc is clearly shown to cause the back and leg pain. Can this also be treated without surgery? In many cases it can if the person is prepared to be limited in activity and continue the basic medical treatment program. Fifty percent of patients with sciatica may improve after 6 weeks.

Full recovery may take more weeks or months. Long-term results suggest that after 4 to 10 years, persons treated with and without surgery are about the same.

Several types of surgery are available to treat those who have ruptured lumbar discs. The ruptured disc can be removed (*discectomy*) by standard surgery techniques. This usually requires being in the hospital for 7 to 10 days. There is a recovery period of weeks to months, depending on the individual situation. Physical therapy and rehabilitation are almost as important as the surgery for full recovery.

Newer techniques include removal of the disc through a very small incision (*percutaneous discectomy*). This allows a much shorter time in hospital, usually only a few days. The success rates are 80 to 90 percent for good relief of pain.

Another method uses injection of a chemical, chymopapain, to "dissolve" the ruptured disc. This is called *chemonucleolysis*. It was more popular a few years ago because an injection seemed to be an easier way to solve the problem. It gives good pain relief in 60 to 80 percent of cases. However, it may have some serious unwanted effects including allergic reaction. If not successful, then surgery may still be needed for treatment of the ruptured disc.

With the treatments available, more than 95 percent of the people with acute back pain are able to find relief and return to their activities. Those who continue to have pain and limitation may need other measures to control what has become chronic pain.

Chronic Back Pain

Chronic back pain occurs when there is no relief after weeks to months of pain. Since most back pain improves, few people experience this pain compared to acute back pain. But these persons are often in constant pain, unable to work and require much medical care.

The pain may not be as intolerable as in early stages of acute back pain, but it is constant and often severely limiting. The pain is usually deep, aching, dull, or burning. It may be felt only in the lower back but commonly travels down one or both legs. Numbness or tingling may be present in the legs.

The constant pain usually affects a person's overall attitude and personality. The pain often prevents sleep. The person becomes more irritable and more difficult to be around. The search for pain relief often leads to the need for stronger pain medications and the use of codeine, propoxyphene (Darvon), or other narcotics. The longer this pattern goes on, the more difficult it becomes to change. With the constant pain, many persons become discouraged and depressed. It is best to perform the testing needed as early as possible to make a reasonable diagnosis of the cause of the pain.

After discussion and examination, one or more of the tests discussed earlier will likely be needed. The computed tomographic scan, magnetic resonance imaging, myelography, bone scan, and other studies may be needed to arrive at a reasonable diagnosis. If the problem is not treatable with surgery, then medical treatment is begun.

Treatment

The basic treatment plan is still the best starting point for treatment as discussed for acute back pain. A regular exercise program is extremely important including twice daily moist heat and exercises. The chances of improvement increase if the program is followed regularly. Those who do not improve almost always are not able to follow a regular program of heat and exercises. More than 90 percent of persons who follow a proper exercise program have some relief of pain.

Because the pain and stiffness have been present for months or longer, it may be difficult to start the exercises at home. We have found it is often easier to begin exercises with a physical therapist. This may even be needed daily. When the person is finally able to accomplish the moist heat and exercises at home twice daily, then visits to the therapist may be needed only occasionally.

Medications Used in Treatment

Medications are used just as in the treatment of acute back pain. The noncortisone anti-inflammatory drugs, the muscle relaxers, and, when necessary, pain medications can be used. Pain medications should be limited to aspirin or acetaminophen if possible. The pain may be long-lasting and the regular use of narcotics for this type of pain increases the chance of dependency.

A group of medications that may give relief in chronic back pain are the antidepressants (Table 6.1). These medications may have an anti-inflammatory effect at lower doses and may directly decrease the pain. Because depression is common in chronic pain, the higher doses used as an anti-depressant may give additional benefit. Other ways to manage chronic back pain are discussed in Chapter 8.

Transcutaneous electrical nerve stimulation (TENS) uses electrodes attached by pads. From 10 to 35 percent of patients with chronic back pain may have good long-term pain relief using TENS. It is safe and relatively inexpensive if it gives adequate relief.

CHAPTER TEN

Advice and Winning Tips

Winning with Arthritis has helped you understand what arthritis is, what type of arthritis you might have, and which treatments are the most effective. There may be no better advice than that given by people who have actually gone through the process. Some persons who are winning with severe arthritis told us what feelings they had, how they coped with their arthritis, and what tips or suggestions they would give to others. This advice is direct from successful managers of arthritis!

How Did You Feel When You Found Out That You Had Arthritis?

Relief

Many persons told us that they felt relief to know that there was a reason for the constant aching, tiredness, and feeling like the "flu." This is a common reaction, especially when joint swelling is not very obvious and especially in the inflammatory types of arthritis. Those who have dealt with rheumatoid arthritis or systemic lupus erythematosus (lupus) certainly know the feeling of tiredness.

Some tell us that it was not exactly a relief because they knew all along that something was wrong to cause such constant stiffness and tiredness.

Discouragement and Despair

On the other hand, some feel discouragement. When the joint swelling and pain are very obvious, the diagnosis is easier. People with severe arthritis said that they were not mentally prepared to cope with the change from an active, independent individual to sudden physical deterioration. The difficulty moving around and the need for assistance in daily activities caused despair at first.

Anger

Why me? I had done my best to fulfill my role in life—why should I be saddled with this disease? Some people feel anger towards their families, their friends, their physicians, or themselves.

Frustration

Many are frustrated at feeling less agile. Difficulty with tasks such as sewing or hammering because the fingers may not always cooperate adds to frustration. At times it may be embarrassing trying to get up from a low or soft chair. Even sexual activity becomes painful and difficult. Personal and family goals might need to be adjusted.

Fear

Fear of what will happen in the future builds. With these limitations, will I have to give up many activities that I now enjoy? What will it be like in one or five years? What will my family do?

Personality Changes

When arthritis is active, pain may be severe. Many told us that they realized they were moody, irritable, and more difficult to get along with. One person describes it as her "Dr. Jekyll and Mr. Hyde" feelings.

How Did You Cope with Your Arthritis?

Acceptance

Most people told us they eventually realized that their arthritis might not go away, that they would have to find a way to cope with it.

Make a Plan to Manage the Arthritis

After acceptance of the arthritis, many people decided they would do whatever was needed to control it. The first step was to learn the facts. When the facts were known, the arthritis usually became much less frightening. They realized that even in severe arthritis there is a good chance to be able to do most of the activities planned for your life with some adjustments.

Relief Again

Once the plan is made, most feel more in control again. There are ways to manage the discomfort. "I then knew that there are things I can do that will influence the course of my disease." Some told us that they taught themselves to be grateful for the good days and to coexist with the discomfort of the bad days. ". . . having lived with the disease for over 16 years, I know it is possible to overcome many things."

What Advice or Tips Would You Give Others with the Disease?

Develop a Good, Strong, Positive Mental Attitude

This may be the most powerful weapon you have to fight back with. It is a slow process but the rewards are wonderful. Some people said:

- "Don't ever give up on what you *can* do."
- "When I get depressed, I try to focus on what I *can* do."
- "I decided it was not going to keep me from doing what I wanted to do."

- "I could adjust and learn to live with it. At first I remember that it was more frightening not knowing what was wrong than actually finding out the diagnosis of rheumatoid arthritis. I realized I could adjust and learn to live with it. I would not allow the arthritis to stop me from living a good and fulfilling life and pursuing my career. These decisions early have kept me going through any hard, frustrating times that have happened."

- "I learned to make adjustments in my career path and lifestyle to accommodate my physical strength. Each job has allowed me to use previously acquired skills to keep my career a success while demanding less of me physically. I am proud of the fact that I have only missed three days of work due to arthritis—when I had a joint replacement in a finger. The trick for me is to get up in the morning no matter how much it hurts, knowing that the pain will get better as the day does on."

- "I fit my medical visits into my own schedule, found time for exercise, and learned my life could go on fairly normally if I was willing to work at it. It is important to realize that you can continue to have a high quality of life. Don't give into the pain, your body will adjust to new pain levels. Most importantly, keep going!"

Don't be afraid to get help from a physician, physical therapist, or counselor. Support is very important. Also make a commitment to follow your treatment with the moist heat, exercises, medications, and whatever else is needed to help. Do this basic treatment plan on good days as well as bad days. Realize that stress can affect your arthritis and work at eliminating stressful situations in your life.

One pianist who developed arthritis in her hands limited her appearances because she worried that it might affect her performance. She did not seek treatment because of the fear of being told to stop the piano. As a result, treatment was delayed and she was quite uncomfortable.

She eventually decided to be evaluated for her hand pain and swelling. She began a regular exercise program, used paraffin baths for heat on the hands, began medication, and has returned to her piano with only minor limitation.

The most common idea among those who are successfully managing their arthritis is that of a *positive mental attitude*. This seems to allow them to continue a regular treatment program. It also helps them minimize their limitations. These people turn arthritis which is terrible into an inconvenience that can be lived with. Simply having a positive attitude seems to increase the chances of a better response.

Another winning idea among those who are winning with arthritis is that of keeping a sense of humor. We were surprised to find that so many successful patients included the importance of a sense of humor.

- "Never lose your ability to laugh."
- "I try to keep a sense of humor about the whole thing. I was asked on vacation why (with arthritis) I stood in cold water in a mountain stream. I said that I can either hurt here or in bed, and I'd rather be here."
- Adaptability is important. Learn to continue activities or make adjustments to get around obstacles due to arthritis.
- "I love to sew. When my arthritis first happened, I stopped sewing. But when I began to sew again, accepting some discomfort and taking a little longer, I became much more satisfied again."

One writer developed arthritis with weakness and deformities in his hands so that he had difficulty using a pen and even typing. He found that adjusting his writing methods using the "soft" touch of a computer keyboard allowed him to resume his work.

One woman with severe arthritis in the hands has difficulty cutting meat with knife and fork. She found a solution when dining out. She now asks the server to have the meat cut into bite-size pieces before it is served.

Many people mentioned the role of stress in their arthritis. Some, but not all, find that in periods of emotional stress their arthritis becomes more active and may have a severe flare up. Their advice is to try to remove the stress or manage it as well as possible while continuing their regular treatment program. (We suggest this plan also, and if the flare up continues, treat the arthritis just as in any other flare up.)

Some people commented on how family and friends reacted to their arthritis. Most found support, but also found that even spouse or family members had some difficulty understanding some things about arthritis. Most often mentioned was the difficulty understanding the severe fatigue, especially in rheumatoid arthritis.

The need for more rest and the lack of endurance for even pleasurable activities may be hard to understand. The lack of obvious signs of sickness is frustrating in some cases. A patient may *feel* much more fatigued and uncomfortable than they look. This can be hard on young families that may require much daily care and direct supervision by the affected adult.

Some people have found helpful ways to follow the basic treatment program. Those who have done the moist heat and exercises regularly and found improvement know that it is necessary to continue. They find that it is best in the long run to make themselves do their exercises on good days as well as bad days, even if it means getting up a few minutes earlier in the morning or staying up a few minutes later at night.

These people also find the fatigue is much less and energy improved when they exercise. Some might suppose that exercise would only cause more tiredness, but more commonly energy improves when exercises are done properly.

Most people who do daily exercises find that when they can't keep up a regular program (when traveling or for other reasons), they don't feel as well. The "old" feelings of pain and stiffness begin to return. Some tell us that their families help them maintain a regular program. This is because they feel and act differently when maintaining a regular treatment program. Families and friends can tell that they feel better when on the regular program.

Most people do *not* like to take medicines. They feel dependent on the medications, even though they realize there is no physical addiction. They do not like the loss of control shown by the need to take medications to function. When they realize that they can help make a difference in the amount of medication needed by maintaining a regular basic treatment plan, it becomes more tolerable. In fact, some people are able to stop medications for periods of time or even permanently after improvement begins. This is more likely to happen if a regular treatment program is followed.

Most people do *not* like the need to see a physician on a regular basis. This also becomes more tolerable when they realize that in most cases more frequent visits are needed when arthritis is active and flaring, but in periods of improved control of arthritis, these physician visits will be needed less often.

Most people who take medications which need regular blood tests or other monitoring do *not* like it. But the benefits of improved control are worth the medications to improve the previous pain, stiffness, and loss of activity. And it is usually understood that treatment must be given safely or the benefits may not be worth the risks, since every medicine has potential unwanted effects. Monitoring medication properly is the best way to prevent complications from treatment.

Most people need to call for advice when something unexplained happens or a new problem appears. When they know what to expect from medications and treatments, a new feeling or sign that doesn't fit is the most common reason for an unscheduled phone call or visit. For example, a fever persisting with no other signs of a simple cold or other virus infection, severe diarrhea lasting more than a few days without other signs of a "bug," and nausea or other stomach discomfort lasting longer than would be expected.

These situations each might represent a serious complication of the underlying condition or might be a serious complication of a medication. Most people feel it is very important to be able to feel comfortable in calling their physician to ask for advice. They prefer to be able to handle the problem over the telephone, but don't mind seeing a physician if needed.

Support Groups

Many people with arthritis enjoy the benefits of a support group, self-help group, or mutual help group. These are small groups with voluntary membership. They help fill the gap in caregiving by professionals and to meet needs not met by institutions. They attempt to deal in many ways with the nonmedical part of arthritis. Members can benefit by giving and receiving help from other members of the group.

These support groups reduce feelings of isolation by looking at a common problem. Some people feel others with the same disease can best understand how they really feel. They no longer feel unique or singled out. When they can share feelings and fears in a safe atmosphere of trust and support, they can feel positive and hopeful again.

These groups offer education about the disease and problem-solving resources. Facts about causes and treatments help others feel more in control. Members can trade tips on managing symptoms. They can also be referred to outside sources for financial, social, psychological and medical help.

- They give mutual support and acceptance. Members can turn to each other for empathy and acceptance through a peer support network. Individuals have help in facing day-to-day struggles with strength from a feeling of all standing together.
- They provide a safe atmosphere for sharing feelings. Because of the trust which usually develops, expressing feelings allows release of tensions and leads to more feelings of peace.
- They can guide members towards a more positive outlook. Members can see others in the same situation, and may learn to accept their problems more readily. They can come to terms with the unfairness of it all, and find more inner strength to cope. This may lead to a feeling of hopefulness and a more positive outlook.

These groups are *not* professional psychotherapy groups. The focus of these groups is to help meet the nonmedical needs of the members. Those who would benefit from further formal psychological or psychiatric treatment should be redirected to better fit their needs.

Support groups can be general and for all arthritis patients. Or, they can be more specialized, dealing with one disease.

Common groups include those for rheumatoid arthritis and systemic lupus erythematosus. The common problems shared, often severe or even life-threatening, make these support groups helpful.

Support groups can be organized by a group of people with a common doctor, a clinic, or by an organization of broader scope such as the Arthritis Foundation or the Lupus Foundation of America. Publicity is usually available free through newspapers and other media. Once begun, the members will guide its course and future as long as it remains useful.

The understanding and support of family members and friends may be helped by education, just as people with arthritis must be educated. The Arthritis Foundation is an excellent source for more information and education of family members. The Arthritis Foundation has a strong national organization with local chapters in most cities. It directly supports research in all areas of arthritis through its efforts and fund raising. The Arthritis Foundation may be contacted at 1314 Spring Street, Atlanta, GA 30309.

The Lupus Foundation of America, Inc. is an excellent source for support and for education of patients and families about Systemic Lupus Erythematosus. There is a strong national chapter with local chapters in most large cities. This is a good resource for information, references about the disease, and referral for specific problems related to lupus. The Lupus Foundation also is an active supporter of research in the causes and treatment of lupus. The address for more information is The Lupus Foundation of America, Inc., 1717 Massachusetts Ave., N.W., Suite 203, Washington, DC 20036.

The Ankylosing Spondylitis Foundation is a national organization with local chapters. It is dedicated to education, support and research in ankylosing spondylitis. It is an excellent resource for further information. The national office can be reached by mail at 511 N. La Cienega Boulevard, Suite 216, Los Angeles, CA 90048.

Sjogren's Syndrome is less common but no less troublesome to its sufferers. Information about current research, current treatments and recent developments can be obtained through Sjogren's Syndrome Foundation, Inc. at 382 Main Street, Port Washington, NY 11050.

The United Scleroderma Foundation can be reached at P. O. Box 350, Watsonville, CA 95077-0350. This organization offers current information regarding education, research, treatments, and latest developments for persons interested in this disease.

The American Association of Retired Persons (AARP) is an active organization dedicated to helping all senior citizens. You can write to the AARP for membership information at 1909 K St. N.W., Washington, DC 20049. With the small yearly membership fee, you will receive a subscription to the magazine *Modern Maturity* which is full of practical advice on retirement, group health insurance, travel, volunteer opportunities, healthcare, and more.

Another organization which is an excellent resource for materials on aging, related diseases, and the rights of mature adults is the National Council on Aging. Their address is 600 Maryland Avenue, S.W., West Wing 100, Washington, DC 20024.

CHAPTER ELEVEN

Questions Asked

Each day we are asked a multitude of questions about arthritis. Questions come from patients, family members and persons who want to find out what can be done to prevent pain and disability from arthritis in the future.

Communication with your physician is important in arthritis. If necessary, we suggest patients write down concerns they may have before the visit so that all questions will be answered. This will make the understanding and treatment of your arthritis more effective.

These are some of the most commonly asked questions.

Q: *A 40-year-old mother of three asks, "I am active and play tennis 3 times a week, but lately when I awake in the morning my thumbs feel stiff and sore. My father has osteoarthritis with a constant problem of pain in his hands. Is this the first sign that I have arthritis? Will I have to stop playing tennis?"*

If the pain and stiffness in the thumbs is persistent over a few months, it is certainly possible that you might be affected by arthritis. Remember that arthritis refers to joint pain, swelling, warmth, or other signs of inflammation. There are other causes of painful hands and thumbs which must be considered such as tendinitis or injury.

After discussion and examination, x-rays and blood tests can help tell whether your problem is arthritis and if it is osteoarthritis. Osteoarthritis is the most common type of arthritis and although it is more standard with people over age 50, it also happens to younger persons, most typically women. When it does, it very commonly involves the joints at the *base of the thumb* or *nearest the fingernails*. It often affects a number of family members, especially women. (See Figure 11.1.)

There may be enough inflammation that osteoarthritis in these situations may appear to be another more severe or destructive type of arthritis. It commonly has a period of inflammation lasting months or years. Then the pain may subside, even though there still may be some swelling.

It is especially important during the period of inflammation to keep the joints as flexible and strong as possible. Then if the osteoarthritis does subside, your joints will still be useful.

Osteoarthritis of this type will mainly affect the hands, but it is not likely to be crippling. Your activities do not have to be

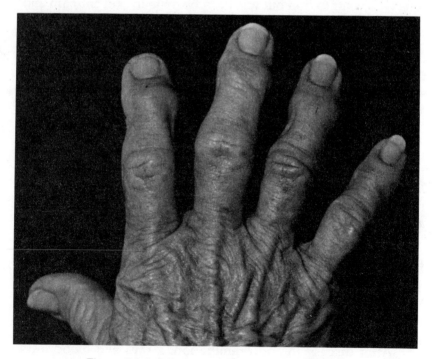

Figure 11.1.   Hand affected by osteoarthritis.

limited, including playing tennis. If you maintain a program of heat and exercises (with medication, if needed) then you will not likely be very limited. The purpose of treatment is to allow you to use the joint, so there are no specific limitations on activity when improvement occurs.

Q: "I work as a copywriter for a local magazine and spend hours at my computer terminal. I am getting concerned because lately during the evening hours, my fingers have a tingling sensation and periodically my fingers go numb during the night. These symptoms go away if I don't type for several days, but come again when I begin my writing. What should I do? Is this arthritis? I love my career and don't see any changes in my job for the near future."

The numbness and tingling you feel, especially in the thumb and nearest two fingers, may be due to pressure around a nerve in the wrist which supplies this area. This is called the median nerve, and the problem may be *carpal tunnel syndrome*. It can also cause weakness in the muscles of the hand. It is usually made worse with increased activity using the wrist and hand. It may awaken you from sleep. It commonly happens while driving a car.

Carpal tunnel syndrome can be caused by arthritis as well as other causes. If other problems are not present, it can be treated with a splint, at times a local injection, or, if needed, by surgery. This should not be a severely limiting problem and should not make you change your career (see page 146).

Q: "I have had arthritis in my hands and knees for a few years. I usually can manage pretty well, but when there is a change in the weather, especially when a cold front or rain comes, I feel much worse. My family tells me this worsening of arthritis is in my head. Is that true?"

Many patients notice a difference in their joint pain and stiffness with weather changes. Some seem to be affected by every change in the weather, and some can never tell a difference. The weather changes which seem to be bothersome to most persons are changes in barometric pressure and humidity. Some are affected by temperature changes. Some feel better in cold weather, some better when it is hot.

Those who are affected may be quite sensitive to the effect of weather changes. It is real, even though it does not affect each person to the same degree. It does not seem to have any other special significance, and is not thought to be a bad or a good sign as far as the arthritis is concerned.

Q: "My 4-year-old daughter has juvenile rheumatoid arthritis. Is this inherited? If we have other children will they also have arthritis? How can we be supportive but not over-protective so she can have as normal a childhood as possible?"

Juvenile rheumatoid arthritis can have a wide range of severity. As discussed on page 35, it can have a form with fever, rash, internal organ disease, with or without prominent joint pain or swelling (the systemic form). The more common forms are those in which the arthritis affects more than 4 joints or the form in which one joint (often the knee) to 4 joints are involved. Each form behaves a little differently from the others.

There has not been any specific evidence that these are inherited diseases or that you need to worry about your next child being affected. Ankylosing spondylitis is a form of arthritis which affects the spine and can affect children (more commonly boys). A higher risk of the possibility of developing this disease can be inherited. However, at this time this fact alone does not usually prevent a couple from having children as planned.

The goal is for children affected by arthritis to lead as normal life as possible. Fortunately, 50 percent or more may have a remission so the prognosis is usually good. Making sure the child keeps a regular exercise program, uses medication when needed, and has proper medical follow up (including eye examinations) are important. We encourage as much activity as the child tolerates. Children usually stay active on their own and don't usually need to be held back. Many children participate in swimming, gymnastics, and lead a quite normal life.

Q: "I am 68 years old and live alone. I have rheumatoid arthritis and am concerned about my ability to continue to do daily living tasks. Is there information available on how to manage such activities as buttons, bathing, opening jars and other such problems when alone?"

The activities of daily living can become difficult in severe arthritis, especially rheumatoid arthritis. Remember to follow the basic treatment program. Also, be sure you are gaining the best possible control of your arthritis with medical treatment.

Your physician or physical therapist can show you a number of items which are very helpful for daily tasks when arthritis is severe. For example, there are simple devices which make it easy to use buttons. Jar openers and devices to help with shoes, dressing, and most other daily needs are available.

There are catalogues which show all of these devices (see references on page 223), many of which are inexpensive but ingenious. If you have trouble locating these items, call your Arthritis Foundation chapter for help.

Q: *"I have taken a NSAID for several days for ankle pain due to an injury. After the third day, I had severe pains in my stomach. Although I felt some relief from the pain in my ankle, I quit taking the medication due to the stomach upset. The upset stomach went away at that time, but what do I do now for the joint pain?"*

You were correct in stopping the NSAID medication. If side effects happen, especially with upset stomach, nausea, abdominal pain or vomiting, then the medication should be stopped at least until you talk to your physician. These could be signs of peptic ulcer disease or other problems which may cause bleeding or other complications.

Even though most persons who take NSAIDS do not have side effects, you should be constantly aware of the possibility of the problems listed on page 51. We suggest that if any new feeling or sign happens which you can't easily explain, then you should check with your physician.

Q: *"I am a 25-year-old woman and have rheumatoid arthritis. I am planning to be married soon and am concerned about the chance of my children having rheumatoid arthritis."*

Over the past few years it has been found that a certain protein which is inherited (called HLA-DR4) is more common in adults with rheumatoid arthritis. This inherited protein in some way increases the chance of developing rheumatoid arthritis. However, of all patients with rheumatoid arthritis, a minority seem to have a number of close family members affected. At this time there are no specific recommendations that patients with rheumatoid arthritis avoid pregnancy because of a high risk of arthritis in the child.

It is usually easier on the mother if the pregnancy is during a time of better control of the arthritis. During pregnancy there is often a spontaneous improvement in the arthritis. After the pregnancy, some women may have a flare up of the arthritis which can usually be treated and controlled.

Q: "I have been out of work due to arthritis. We are barely able to live on my wife's salary. I was wondering if there was any government relief fund that I could turn to for financial help?"

Social Security provides basic protection against the loss of family income due to the disability of a major income earner. Under Social Security, the definition of disability is related to the ability to work. A person is considered disabled and receives benefits for a severe physical or mental impairment or combination of impairments that prevents work for a year or more. The work can be any gainful work, not just the previous occupation. This is discussed in an easy-to-understand way in *The 50+ Wellness Program* (McIlwain, et al., John Wiley & Sons, Inc., 1989). You can also call your Social Security office for more information.

Q: "I am a 28-year-old woman and was recently told that I have systemic lupus erythematosus. Is there anything I can do to avoid relapses and worsening of my disease?"

Lupus can cause a wide variety of problems, ranging from very mild and nonlimiting to life threatening internal organ disease such as kidney disease or heart disease. It would be a good idea to review with your physician where your specific situation fits compared to other patients with lupus. Also, understand what, if any, internal organ involvement there may be.

Follow the basic treatment program and know how often you need medical follow-up to be sure no new problems develop. Some patients with mild disease need only occasional visits to their physician. Relapses may not be preventable and will often happen at the most inconvenient time. During periods of more active disease you will probably need more frequent contact with your physician to allow medications to be adjusted.

The best way to prevent progression of disease is to continue regular medical follow-up, to treat the flares and internal organ problems if they happen. This is a disease in which we don't always have control over disease flares or progression. However, there are many very effective medications now available so that most patients can manage their disease successfully.

Q: *"My 65-year-old mother has osteoporosis, which was found after she recently fell and broke her hip. What is the difference between osteoporosis and osteoarthritis? What can I do to prevent further deterioration of her bones?"*

Osteoporosis is actually a different problem than osteoarthritis. Osteoporosis is thinning of the bones so that eventually the bones become weak enough to break. It is most common in women, especially after menopause, but happens in men as well. The most common bones which break are the hip, the spine, and the wrist. In older persons a broken hip can be a devastating problem. Up to 20 percent of these persons may die within the first year.

Osteoporosis can be treated. There are medications and other treatments which can slow the thinning of the bones and help make them stronger. The goal of treatment is to prevent the next fracture. Your mother should talk with her physician about the treatments available. You may want to read a book which explains the prevention and treatment of osteoporosis in easily understood language (*Osteoporosis: Prevention, Management, Treatment* listed in the references on page 224).

Osteoarthritis is the most common type of arthritis. It is discussed on page 21. A person may have either osteoporosis, osteoarthritis, or both. Each can be treated without conflict with the other treatment.

Q: *"My grandfather has severe arthritis. His hands and fingers are swollen and bent. How did this happen? Can he be helped at this point? How can I prevent this from happening to me?"*

The arthritis you describe in your grandfather could be severe osteoarthritis, especially if it only involves the fingers. It could also be rheumatoid arthritis or other more serious type of arthritis. The swelling and pain come from inflammation in the joints.

In rheumatoid arthritis, the joints remain swollen over a period of time, usually years, the structures that hold the joint together (the tendons, ligaments, and muscles) become "looser" and less effective. This allows the joints to become deformed. In some types of arthritis there is actually destruction of portions of the bones which contributes to deformity.

There is treatment available. The *active* arthritis (the swelling, warmth) can usually be treated with a basic treatment program and medications to improve pain and stiffness. This usually also improves the use of the joints.

The deformity from the arthritis which has been present over the years may not be as reversible. If there is improvement but deformities still cause limitation, then he could consider surgery for the arthritis. He should talk with his physician, since it is almost never too late to have some improvement in pain and use of the joints.

You should not be alarmed about getting severe arthritis as an inherited problem, although it depends in part on what type of arthritis your grandfather is found to have. You may want to watch for warning signs of arthritis. If you have persistent pain, stiffness or swelling in the joints then have it checked. Deformities in arthritis are much more effectively *prevented* with proper treatment than reversed after they happen.

Q: "My husband is 50 years old. He has always been athletic, and plays golf and tennis regularly. He has not played as often lately because his right shoulder has been painful. Does this mean he must stop his activities? This would change his life as his sports are a nice source of stress release."

If your husband feels well otherwise and has pain only in one shoulder, it is actually most likely that his problem is bursitis or tendinitis around the shoulder. This can be very painful and is usually made worse by activities such as golf and tennis. However, it is very treatable and usually responds to a basic treatment program of heat, exercises, medication and at times a local injection.

Bursitis or tendinitis around the shoulder is usually not permanent and should not be severely limiting if treated. In fact, if there is not a good response then there should be further evaluation to be sure no other problem is present. Your husband should have the shoulder checked to see what is needed to solve the problem. Then he will probably be able to resume his activities.

Q: "I am a 45-year-old man and have been running 15 miles a week for years. It is the best stress release I know and I love it. Lately my knees have been stiff which has made running more uncomfortable. Help!"

If no other joints are affected and if the stiffness has been present for a number of months, it is possible that you may have early arthritis in the knees. If so, the most likely type is probably osteoarthritis, although it is possible that other problems might be present.

If proper evaluation shows that the problem is osteoarthritis, then a basic treatment program should be started, emphasizing exercises for the muscles which support the knees. After a period of weeks to months there should be improvement in the stiffness in the knees.

For the long term, it might be a good idea to think about adding bicycle or swimming to your exercise program. These would be excellent cardiovascular exercises but would put much less stress on your knees. You may be able to prolong your years of running in this way. If you continue to use only running as exercise at this time, you should continue an exercise program to improve the support for the knees.

Q: A 43-year-old electrician asks, "Over the past few months my right elbow has become painful when I work. Now I have trouble using my right arm. My hand grip is weak and it even hurts to shake hands. What can be done?"

If no other joints or areas are painful, and if you have not injured the elbow, then one of the most likely problems is tendinitis around the elbow. This goes by other names such as "tennis elbow," "little league elbow," and others. The problem is inflammation of the tendon that attaches one of the muscles of the lower arm to the elbow. Each time the muscle is used (as in handgrip, squeezing with the hand, throwing a ball or using a screwdriver) it pulls the tendon and causes pain.

This is often caused by repetitive use or movements using the muscle, especially if an excess amount of use is done over a short time. The treatment is as outlined on page 25 with the basic treatment program. Temporarily avoiding those movements which hurt will help, although this is often not possible. We suggest the use of twice daily moist heat with an ice pack immediately after use of the elbow. There are specific exercises which can be done to help prevent this from returning.

Q: A 45-year-old woman asks, "I am worried that I may be developing arthritis. I have had severe pain in my thumb over the past few months. Now I can't even pinch or make a fist because my thumb seems to catch and lock in one position. What should I do?"

If the main problem is in one thumb, and the thumb "catches" when you bend it, your problem may be what is called a *"trigger finger or snapping thumb."* This is caused by inflammation of the sheath around the tendon which moves the thumb. The inflammation causes swelling so that the tendon moves one way more easily than the other. This causes it to be painful and "catch" on movement.

This may happen in arthritis of several different types or may happen alone. The trigger finger can be injected locally which usually gives relief. If not, then surgery can correct the problem.

Q: A 49-year-old painter asks, "Over the past 6 months I have had pain and stiffness in my shoulders, knees, and wrists. It has become hard to "get going" in the morning, and my energy is terrible. I am afraid this will make it hard to continue my business. I have to be able to climb, use a roller and paint to make a living. What can I do?"

You should definitely see your physician to find out what is causing your problem. There are many medical problems which may mimic arthritis. If arthritis is found to be present then one of the possibilities is rheumatoid arthritis or other inflammatory arthritis.

If proper diagnosis is made then a basic treatment program can begin. There is usually improvement over a period of weeks to 2 months. If there is not adequate improvement and rheumatoid arthritis is found to be the problem then there is another group of medications which helps to control the disease, the "suppressive" drugs.

It is most important that you do not give up and that you realize that you do *not* have to just live with it. A high priority should be to keep you working, which can usually be done with treatment.

Q: A 50-year-old man asks what to do about severe pain and swelling in an ankle. He travels frequently and for the past week has been unable to drive due to pain in his right ankle. He had similar attacks 3 and 6 months ago in his left ankle. Each time it went away after about 1 week.

This man probably has acute arthritis in the right ankle. The treatment depends on the cause. After discussion and examination, a good way to find the cause of the arthritis is to examine a sample of joint fluid from the ankle. This is a simple procedure done with local anesthetic. Examination of the joint fluid in this situation under a special microscope (a polarizing microscope) often finds crystals which make the diagnosis of gout.

Gout usually causes acute arthritis in the first toe, ankle, or knee but can affect other joints. It is treatable and when medication is taken regularly, it is almost always controlled so that there are no attacks of arthritis at all. If not treated, it can progress to a disabling arthritis. Gout is one kind of arthritis you don't have to live with.

Q: A 65-year-old man says, "I am retired but very active. I volunteer 20 hours weekly working with children. For 3 months I have had terrible pain and stiffness, first in my shoulders, now in my hips and thighs. I have trouble lifting my arms to comb my hair because of the pain. The stiffness in the morning lasts until noon. My energy is poor. At night it hurts to turn over in bed. I have never felt so bad. What can I do?"

The pain you describe is definitely not "old age," and is *not* very typical of the most common kind of arthritis, osteoarthritis, which comes on gradually and less often affects the shoulders in this way. It is more typical of polymyalgia rheumatica.

Polymyalgia rheumatica often strikes otherwise healthy persons, with the cause unknown. It causes severe pain and stiffness in the shoulders, arms, hips and thighs. It causes severe stiffness in the morning and usually very uncomfortable nights.

If no other medical problems are found to be present then there is usually a dramatic response to a low dose of prednisone or other cortisone derivative. Usually within days there is excellent improvement in the pain and stiffness. Then the dose of prednisone is gradually lowered and stopped after a period which is variable, from a few months to 2 years or more.

You should see your physician since there is good treatment available. It is also important to be sure no other medical problems co-exist with the polymyalgia rheumatica.

Q: A 15-year-old girl asked, "I am a dancer. I've been dancing since I was 7. My left knee began to be painful and swollen 4 months ago even though I didn't hurt it. Then my other knee and wrists started hurting a few weeks ago. My mother says I must stop dancing. What can I do?"

This girl was actually seen over a year ago. After discussion and examination, some x-rays and blood tests helped in making the diagnosis of juvenile rheumatoid arthritis. She began a basic treatment program of moist heat, exercises and anti-inflammatory medication. There was improvement after a few months and she gradually increased her activity. She now dances with only occasional pain and stiffness in the knees.

Q: A 66-year-old lady asks, "I have had pain and stiffness in my knees and back once in a while for years, but never let it bother me. Over the past year, I have had more and more trouble. Now I have trouble walking even with a walker due to pain in the knees and back. I was told I have arthritis. What should I do?"

The pain you are feeling in the knees and back may well be due to arthritis, and it may be osteoarthritis, the most common type. It is most common in the joints that bear weight over the years, such as the knees, hips, and often happens in the lower back. Of course, there are other causes of this pain. If present, these other problems can be found by your physician. X-rays and other tests should be able to help decide.

If it is osteoarthritis, then a basic treatment program of moist heat, exercises and medications should be started. If there is not adequate improvement over a period of a few months with this program, then it might be a good idea to consider the possibility of surgery.

If the knee pain becomes the most limiting problem then surgery might offer improvement in pain and ability to walk. If osteoarthritis in the back is the main source of pain, surgery may not be as helpful. In this case, let your physician and orthopedic surgeon give you advice. If the basic treatment program gives enough improvement, avoid surgery. If there is not enough improvement, see what surgery has to offer so that you can weigh the benefits and risks in your own situation.

Q: A 52-year-old lady was seen because of severe pain in the right hip. She worried that she might have arthritis, and was concerned that the pain was severe enough to think about surgery. The pain was so severe that she had trouble sitting in a chair or lying on her right side at night.

After discussion and examination, x-rays showed only mild osteoarthritis in the right hip. The problem turned out to be *bursitis* around the hip. This bursitis can cause severe pain and may be incapacitating. It can come on suddenly or gradually, and can even happen along with other arthritis.

Even though the pain can be severe, the cause is not as severe. The bursitis is treated with a basic treatment program of moist heat, exercises, and medication. At times a local injection is needed. This lady did well and after a few weeks had no further pain in the hip. She has continued her regular exercise program.

Q: A 50-year-old travel agent was seen after 1 year of aching and stiffness "all over." She had pain in the arms, legs, neck and back which was constant. She felt very stiff in the mornings. She was constantly tired. She had trouble sleeping at night and often awakened with pain. She had been to several clinics over the year, and her work was becoming more difficult.

After discussion and examination as well as some other tests and x-rays, this lady was found to have fibrositis. This also is called fibromyalgia. The cause is not known, and it does not cause deformities, but it results in severe pain and stiffness. Most persons with fibrositis seem to be able to do their daily tasks, but with much discomfort.

If no other problems are present, the treatment for fibrositis includes a basic treatment program of moist heat, exercises and medication. Although there is no cure, the fibrositis usually becomes manageable. This lady improved over a period of 6 months and now continues a regular exercise program.

Q: A 25-year-old man was recently seen because of back pain. He had pain and stiffness in the lower back for over 8 years. It had gradually worsened. On awakening in the morning, the back was stiff for about 2 hours, but improved as he became more active. He had milder aching in the shoulders and hips. He noticed more pain when sitting at his desk in his office for prolonged periods.

This man was found to have ankylosing spondylitis after discussion, examination, and x-rays which showed typical changes in the lower back and sacroiliac joints. He began a basic treatment program and over a few months noticed improvement in pain and stiffness. He found that his energy improved as well. He continues with a regular exercise program and a non-cortisone anti-inflammatory drug (NSAID).

Q: A 63-year-old grandmother asks, "I have arthritis in my hands and knees. I am confused because some of my friends tell me to use heat, and some tell me I should use ice. Which is it?"

Both of your friends may be correct. Moist heat helps to make the joints and muscles more comfortable and relaxed. This allows easier and more effective exercises.

However, ice may be effective for some persons, and some do best if they alternate ice packs with moist heat. Whichever is most effective for you is acceptable. Remember that the moist heat should not be hot enough to be uncomfortable or burn the skin. And the ice should be used in a bag, not directly on the skin.

Q: A 55-year-old lady asks, "I have a copper bracelet my grandmother gave me. She wore it to help her arthritis. She also told me to drink vinegar and honey mixed in water. Are these true treatments for arthritis?"

Copper bracelets have been used for many years as a remedy for arthritis. It is thought that the copper is absorbed through the skin and in some way helps the arthritis. Although this is not proven, it is not harmful and if you feel that it helps, it doesn't hurt to try.

Vinegar and honey mixed with water is a folk remedy. It is believed that there is not enough acid production, which makes arthritis more likely. The vinegar and honey are to help the body in its acid production. If you feel it helps and you use moderate amounts, this should not be harmful although you should check with your physician to be sure it is safe for you. However, there is no evidence that it works in arthritis.

Some remedies are appealing because they appear much easier than the need for the work of twice daily moist heat, exercises, and medication. If you use these, try to set a time limit in which you can judge whether they have helped.

The role of diet (which may be important) along with other non-standard treatments are discussed in Chapter 7.

Q: I have been overweight for years, and my knees and back recently began to be painful and stiff. I was told that I have arthritis in my back and knees and need to lose weight to help. Was my arthritis caused by being overweight all these years?

The most likely type of arthritis in this situation is probably osteoarthritis in the lumbar spine and in the knees. This is most commonly the result of "wear-and-tear" changes on the joint cartilage over the years. It can also happen after injuries, such as an auto accident or athletic injuries.

There is some controversy about whether excess weight actually causes osteoarthritis. Some research has shown that osteoarthritis is more common in persons who are overweight (obese). On the other hand, some researchers have found that it may aggravate arthritis already present, but are less sure that it actually causes the arthritis. When the true causes of osteo-arthritis and other types of arthritis are known, this question will be able to be answered more completely.

From a practical standpoint, a person who has arthritis of any type, especially in the joints that bear weight—the knees, feet, ankles, hips, and back—can help themselves by controlling their body weight. Less weight and stress on the joints may help to decrease the pain. Those who successfully lose weight usually notice some improvement in joint pain as well. It is one more action (just as moist heat, exercises, medication), that can help in the control of pain.

CHAPTER TWELVE

Future Treatment

What new treatments do the 34 million Americans dealing with arthritis have to look forward to in the future? Eventually researchers will be able to tell the causes of many types of arthritis. It is even possible that some causes of serious arthritis will be found to be due to infection. This was the case with Lyme arthritis, which is now treatable. Until then, newer medications and treatments must be tried until we find the most effective possible treatment with the least side effects.

Breakthrough Treatments?

More noncortisone anti-inflammatory drugs (NSAIDS) may become available in the near future. Even though they are not dramatic breakthroughs, these new additions increase the chance that more people will experience improvement in arthritis without side effects. Many of these medications are available earlier through participation in clinical trials. Participating in a clinical trial with these new medications offers a chance to receive the newer treatment with close medical supervision.

Other medications are being developed that decrease inflammation by decreasing the activity of the proteins that act as "messengers" to direct cells to cause more inflammation. This might attack the inflammation of arthritis at a more basic level.

219

One new treatment that may become available is a medication which is injected into a joint called *superoxide dismutase*. This often gives improvement in pain and swelling with few side effects. Since it is not a cortisone derivative, the side effects of cortisone treatment are avoided. This drug has been used so far mainly in osteoarthritis of the knees.

Other possible medications in osteoarthritis in the future may include drugs that attempt to protect or rebuild the joint cartilage. So far, none has proven effective without side effects. In rheumatoid arthritis, there is some early research attempting to create hope for a vaccine for prevention of the disease. This is still in a very preliminary stage.

Surgery and Joint Replacement

Treatment with surgery in osteoarthritis and rheumatoid arthritis will likely continue to improve. Just as total hip replacement improved over the past 10 years, total knee replacement has improved rapidly in the past 5 years. This has given more people, especially older people, the opportunity for improvement in pain and activity. Hopefully, progress will continue for surgery in other joints in osteoarthritis and rheumatoid arthritis.

The Future for Rheumatoid Arthritis

In rheumatoid arthritis, the addition of new noncortisone anti-inflammatory drugs may offer improved control of pain and stiffness. Several newer drugs that are not in this group but which seem to suppress the arthritis are now in testing stages. Some medications that are effective for arthritis are still limited by side effects, such as one called cyclosporin. If ways can be found to give these drugs safely, more people will benefit. Also, newer derivatives of these drugs might later offer similar improvement without such serious side effects.

In severe rheumatoid arthritis, the use of more than one suppressive drug (Table 4.9) at the same time may be more common in the future. These drugs have usually been used alone.

Some researchers have found that a lower dose of more than one drug may be more effective than the standard higher doses of a single drug. It is hoped that the lower doses will allow fewer serious side effects. However, until it is clear how effective these combinations are, most will remain experimental.

A low dose of radiation to the body has been used for severe rheumatoid arthritis. This has given improvement which lasts 6 to 12 months and may extend up to 4 years in some patients. However, there are side effects including serious infections. There is also a concern about the possibility of the development of cancer in later years. This treatment also remains experimental.

Attacking the Inflammation of Arthritis

Researchers are developing proteins called monoclonal antibodies that attack or block the action of some of the cells that trigger inflammation. If these can be improved, it might be possible to "turn off" inflammation of arthritis before it starts. This treatment will likely be at least a few years away.

All of these treatments are experimental and are reserved for people who have not responded to other available treatments. Your physician can keep you updated on the latest developments and available effective treatments for arthritis.

Suggestions for Further Reading

Catalogues for Assistive Devices

Adaptability Catalogue
P.O. Box 515
Colchester, CT 06415-0515

Enrichments for Better Living Catalogue
P.O. Box 579
Hinscale, IL 60521-9842

Professional Healthcare Catalogue
Fred Sammons, Inc.
Burr Ridge, IL 60521

Books and Articles

Deboskey, D. S., J. M. Engle, and T. W. Oleson (1989) *Pain: Making Life Livable* (Tampa: Deboskey and Associates).

McCarty, D. J., ed. (1987) *Arthritis and Allied Conditions* (Philadelphia: Lea & Febiger).

McIlwain, H. H., D. F. Bruce, J. C. Silverfield, and M. C. Burnette (1988) *Osteoporosis: Prevention, Management, Treatment* (New York: John Wiley).

McIlwain, H. H., L. F. Steinmeyer, D. F. Bruce, R. E. Fulghum, and R. G. Bruce (1989) *The 50+ Wellness Program* (New York: John Wiley).

Physician's Desk Reference (1990) (Oradell, N.J: Edward R. Barnhart. Medical Economics Company).

Schumacher, H. R., ed. (1988) *Primer on the Theumatic Diseases* (Atlanta: The Arthritis Foundation).

Index